Early Reviews of Plague Legends:

Professionals, students and all medical history buffs will be indebted to Socrates Litsios' new *book Plague Legends: from the Miasmas of Hippocrates to the Microbes of Pasteur* for providing an easy access to a treasure of information. This finely crafted, scholarly book traces the long 2000 years of western civilization during which philosophy, literature, and the arts flourished but medical science remained a confused, often dangerous, body of ignorance. Litsios' book presents an expert account of what the discovery of microbes and their pathogenic potentials meant to human health.

Robert S. Desowitz, PhD, DSc (Lond.)
Emeritus Professor of Tropical Medicine and Medical Microbiology, University of Hawaii
Adjunct Professor of Epidemiology, University of North Carolina at Chapel Hill

Plague Legends is a fascinating contribution to the history of medicine. Its novelty lies in a delicate interweaving of concepts of disease derived from theological beliefs and those based on what would be regarded – even in contemporary terms – as scientific evidence. ...

Litsios' profiles and interpretations of the 18th and 19th century outbreaks of bubonic plague, smallpox, tuberculosis, yellow fever, cholera, and malaria are masterful. Indeed, anyone who wants to understand the complex evolution of ideas pertaining to the major diseases of past centuries and their relationship to evolving levels of evidence, linked to measurement techniques, would be well-advised to read this book and independently track down original sources....

The treatment of the emergence of Public Health in the 18th and 19th centuries in response to the evidence that poverty and disease went hand-in-hand is succinct and to the point. This history seems to be almost invisible in the modern literature focused on inverse associations between social class and health. *Plague Legends* provides a much needed institutional perspective on this topic. The entire book would be a very useful required volume in courses on the history of medicine. Perhaps more importantly, it should be read and discussed by students in schools of public health, where a deeper understanding of the origins of Public Health as a profession and as a broad set of academic topics would be highly desirable.

The author, Socrates Litsios, while claiming to be an amateur historian displays all the characteristics of a practiced professional. His previous book, *The Tomorrow of Malaria*, clearly displays the author's depth of thought, thoroughness of investigation, and engaging writing style. *Plague Legends* continues this tradition....

Burton Singer, Ph.D.

Charles and Marie Robertson Professor of Public and International Affairs, Princeton University

Plague Legends

From the Miasmas of Hippocrates

To the Microbes of Pasteur

Socrates Litsios

Science & Humanities Press

Chesterfield, Missouri, USA

Library of Congress Cataloging-in-Publication Data

Litsios, Socrates, 1937-
  Plague legends : from the miasmas of Hippocrates to the microbes of Pasteur / Socrates Litsios.
     p. ; cm.
Includes bibliographical references and index.
  ISBN 1-888725-33-8
  1. Medicine--History. 2. Germ theory of disease--History.
  [DNLM: 1. Communicable Diseases--history. 2. Communicable Disease Control--history. 3. Disease Outbreaks--history. 4. Plague--history.
WC 11.1 L776p 2001] I. Title.
  R131 .L56 2001
  610'.9--dc21   2001002147

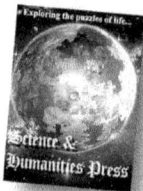

Science & Humanities Press

PO Box 7151

Chesterfield, MO 63006-7151

(636) 394-4950

http :www.sciencehumanitiespress.com

E-mail: publisher@sciencehumanitiespress.com

Plague Legends

From the Miasmas of Hippocrates

To the Microbes of Pasteur

Socrates Litsios

Contents

Prologue...1

Introduction 3

PART I - PRE 18th CENTURY HISTORY 7

Ancient roots of 18th century medicine 7

The Hippocratic Legacy 7

The Galenic Legacy 11

Ancient Medicine Shaped by Christianity..17

Decline of Galenism and the Rise of New Schools of Medicine...............21

The Revolt of Paracelsus 23

Galen's Anatomy Revisited by Vesalius 29

Harvey's Explorations of the Heart and Blood 32

Paracelsians and the Iatrochemical School of Medicine.......................36

Boyle's Corpuscles and the Iatrophysical School of Medicine 43

Return to the Hippocratic Bedside 46

On the Origin of Epidemics 51

Neo-Platonic, Religious and Other 'Occult' Influences 51

Germs of Contagion - The Path Least Taken 64

On the Epidemic Constitution of the Atmosphere 71

PART II - DISEASE PROFILES..77

Disease Profiles..77

Plague...78

Smallpox...80

Tuberculosis...82

Diphtheria 84

Scarlet Fever...87

Malaria..88

Influenza...90

Typhus...92

Yellow Fever 94

Cholera..95

Typhoid 98

Epidemic Puerperal Fever...99
Part III - 18th and 19th CENTURY HISTORY 101
    18th Century - A Kind of Status Quo Reigns 101
        Plague in Marseilles: 1720-22...101
        England Awaits the Plague 105
        Tuberculosis - The Ignored Ideas of Benjamin Marten 114
        Cotton Mather Battles Smallpox 118
        Diphtheria in the American Colonies: 1736-40 122
        Malaria in the Roman Campagna 125
        Typhus in England..128
        Influenza - The Views of Arbuthnot and Webster 132
        Yellow Fever in Philadelphia: 1793 136
        Rush's Doctrine of the Unity of Fevers 141
        Webster's Views on the Origin of Yellow Fever 147
    19th Century - Recognition of Disease Specificity.................................153
        Broussais Uses Pathological Anatomy to Show All Fevers to Be the Same 154
        Distinguishing Typhus from Typhoid Fever 160
        Bretonneau Establishes the Specificity of Diphtheria........................166
        Yellow Fever in Europe- To Quarantine or Not? 170
        Cholera Reaches the New World..175
        Apparent Water, Soil and Air Sources of the Malarial Fever 191
        Epidemic Puerperal Fever - A Hand or An Air Borne Disease? 198
        Pasteur Takes on Spontaneous Generation...205
        The Disease Causation Postulates of Koch..211
        Microbial Approach to Public Health 216
Epilogue...229
Acknowledgements 235
Illustration Credits 236
Further Reading..237
Index..247

List of Illustrations

The Four Humors 6

Hippocrates 7

Galen 11

The inluence of the zodiac signs on the human body 18

Protective Amulet 20

Paracelsus 23

Vesalius performing dissection 28

Circulation of the blood 35

Jean Baptiste van Helmont 39

The Spirit of Sulphur 41

Ficino Translation of page from Hermes Trismegistus 49

Preparation and administration of Guaiac wood 55

Enemies Invading the Fortress of Health by Robert Fludd 59

Hieronimus Fracastorius 66

Plague doctor. The "beak" contained fragrant substances 74

The Quarantine Question 76

The Royal Touch 83

La Peste dans la ville de Marseille 104

Plague in 1665 106

Antoni van Leeuwenhoek 115

La Vaccine en Voyage 122

An allegory of malaria 127

Fan on top of Newgate prison 132

Benjamin Rush on blood-letting 146

At The Gates 152

Leech gatherers 159

Le Docteur Bretonneau 166

Yellow fever in Barcelona 171

Cholera in Paris 179

Drake's Poster for the Cure of Cholera 180

Snow's map of Soho 184

Drake's Systematic Treatise 192

Puerpural septicemia: Semmelweis' statistics 200

Pasteur 204

Robert Koch 213

Preparation of rat poison during plague campaign 226

Dedicated to the Memory

of a dear friend and colleague

Kenneth Eugene Mott

(1939-1997)

Prologue

The most fascinating objective has been the history of ideas, the slow and gradual evolution of human thought. How did the leaders of science really visualize a given problem in a given century, what was their solution and what were the reasons which dictated that solution? (Winslow)

The idea of writing this book grew on me slowly. I date its inception, at least in its 'germ' form, to when I first read Charles-Edward A. Winslow's *The Conquest of Epidemic Disease* in 1995. It was there where I first encountered the colorful characters of Benjamin Rush and Max von Pettenkofer, two legendary personalities whose disease theories were so strikingly new to me as to make me realize how ignorant I was of the richness of beliefs concerning the origin of epidemic disease before the reality of the microbial world came into being.

Rush is classified as one of, if not the, leading physician in America at the end of the 18th century. He is also known for his 'heroic' use of bloodletting to cure disease, which has been said to have caused more deaths than the French Revolution and the Napoleonic Wars combined! Pettenkofer too gets a bad historical press, although he is recognized as one of the leading German hygienists of the 19th century. History books, short of space, tell us only about his having deliberately drunk a culture of cholera bacillus, often without even bothering to inform the reader why anyone would commit such an apparently suicidal act.

Both Rush and Pettenkofer are often portrayed as medical anomalies, lacking any sense. Yet Winslow, for good reasons, invests heavily in telling both their stories, Rush's in connection with the 1793 yellow fever epidemic in Philadelphia, and Pettenkofer's in connection with the series of cholera pandemics that struck Europe during the 19th century. We learn how both evolved epidemic causation theories that were fully consistent with earlier thinking whose roots trace back to Hippocrates.

Despite Winslow's extensive accounting of different theories from antiquity to the 20th century, I still did not have a clear picture of how they vied with each other, i.e. why did some believe in one theory while others preferred another. At that point I realized that by writing a book I could hopefully come to that understanding and in the process explain these theories in simpler and more accessible terms.

Plague Legends

It was only when I had completed the first draft that I ran across references to Marsilio Ficino, an ordained priest with some medical training who is best known for his translations of Plato from Greek to Latin in the 1460s. Although Winslow makes several brief references to Ficino's plague treatise, he does not refer to how Ficino's translations of the legendary figure of Hermes Trismegistus led Ficino, followed by other physicians in the 16th and 17th centuries, to incorporate 'Hermetic' ideas in their medical writings. At this point, the goals of my book became a little more ambitious; I wanted to understand how religious beliefs influenced medical theories of epidemics, an orientation rather lacking in the work of Winslow (who concentrated on "leaders of science"), and many other medical historians who have written about disease.

By now the reader may have guessed that I am not a professional historian. While I don't think this lessens my enthusiasm for the subject in any way, it is a handicap. Not only do I not know Latin and other languages that would have allowed me to explore original texts, amateurs are always at greater risk of being taken in by the historical misreading and exaggeration of others and introducing some themselves. Hopefully these risks are compensated for by whatever fresh point of view I have been able to bring to this subject.

If readers get as much pleasure out of this book as I had in writing it, which I truly hope proves to be the case, they will be additionally pleased to learn that the literature covering this subject is vast and mostly accessible. Some suggestions are given in the Further Reading section.

Introduction

*Please sir, don't legends always have a basis in fact? ... 'Well,' said Professor Binns slowly, 'yes, one could argue that, I suppose.' ... However, the legend of which you spoke is such a very **sensational**, even **ludicrous** tale ...' (from J.K. Rowling's Harry Potter and the Chamber of Secrets)*

Legend is a wonderfully ambivalent term. A legend may sometimes have no basis in fact, but more often than not it is built on a mixture of fact and fiction, both of which might contain "sensational" and even "ludicrous" elements. Even real figures of legendary stature rarely escape having some fictitious tale woven into their biography.

Both Hippocrates and Pasteur are of legendary stature. But whereas factual microbes account for much of Pasteur's fame, "miasmas" are strictly fictitious; it is not for them that Hippocrates owes his current fame. Fictitious as they are, however, miasmas dominated the world of epidemics up until the time that microbes came to be accepted as real disease-causing agents. Today some might find miasma-related legends somewhat ludicrous, but their place and importance in history cannot be denied.

Hippocrates used the word miasma to express the idea of a contaminated atmosphere that could give rise to epidemics. In time miasmas were joined by disease-carrying demons, wind-borne morbific matter, and countless other ways of identifying the mysterious nature of a diseased atmosphere. Never far from any of these explanations, however, was Gods' punishment.

Major epidemics were nearly always seen as a form of divine judgement. They provided religious and medical authorities with a convenient opportunity to identify their foes. Thus, the plague epidemic in Munster in Westphalia in 1550 was seen as God's punishment for the heretical activities of the Anabaptists and London's 1665 plague was due to the government having allowed Thomas Hobbes, an atheist, to return there following a long exile in France. Where there were no designated targets, as such, the sinful populace as a whole was always available to be blamed.

Religious factors played a crucial role in shaping medical beliefs and practices well through the 17th century. Religious beliefs constrained as well as motivated certain lines of argument concerning what the epidemic-causing process might be. When the Church was more tolerant towards Neo-Platonic beliefs, during a brief period in the 16th and 17th centuries, many physicians rallied around occult disease theories of the most fantastic kind. These beliefs were the source material for some of the more "sensational" legends of the time.

Many medical history books give short shrift to the legends rooted in Neo-Platonic and other occult ideas. There is almost an embarrassed silence surrounding such a personality as Robert Fludd, for example. Other legendary figures, such as Paracelsus and van Helmont, who also were deeply involved in similar mystical philosophy, generally find a place in history books because their influence and accomplishments are simply too important to be overlooked. However, little attention is given to their 'philosophical' notions.

History books can and do distort on occasion by over exaggerating the importance of a certain personality, attempting to create a modern legend as it were. Winslow, says of Fracastoro, for example, that his "*philosophical statement of the contagionistic theory of disease (was) a mountain peak in the history of etiology perhaps unequalled by any other writer between Hippocrates and Pasteur.*" Fracastoro wrote about "germs" in the 16th century but only achieved great fame during his lifetime as a poet and a learned physician. And about Sydenham, the English Hippocrates, Winslow judges that "*his almost complete neglect of contagion as a practical factor in the spread of epidemic disease and his major stress upon the metaphysical factor of epidemic constitution held back epidemiological progress for two hundred years.*" Sydenham lived some one hundred and fifty years after Fracastoro, and while it is true that he was influential in determining the direction that medical education would take in the 18th century, he was not alone in his neglect of 'contagion' as a factor in the spread of disease.

The book is divided into three parts. Part I covers history up to Sydenham, i.e. up until the end of the 17th century. Part II introduces the specific epidemic diseases that are touched upon in this book. By understanding how each epidemic disease differs, the reader can better appreciate the epidemiological puzzle they presented scientists of the 18th and 19th centuries. Part III picks up the history of plague legends, covering these two centuries. Part III differs in approach from that taken in Part I. To begin with, more attention is given to specific major disease outbreaks, especially those of yellow fever and cholera, two diseases not known in Europe before the 18th century. Also, Part III uses each example to review relevant past histories, sometimes taking the reader back to earlier centuries. On several occasions a forward look is made to the early years of the 20th century to better portray the impact of the microbial basis of disease upon public health thinking and practice.

The short epilogue that concludes the book is a reflection on the fact that microbes are still with us and public health is at best fighting a holding action. Part of the failure to control plague diseases better than we have is due to the fact that public health in the 19th century developed along lines that were somewhat antagonistic to the new science of bacteriology. Although this is not a major objective of this book, it is hoped that the reader will come to realize that something important was lost when microbes were seen to be the end-all of disease thinking.

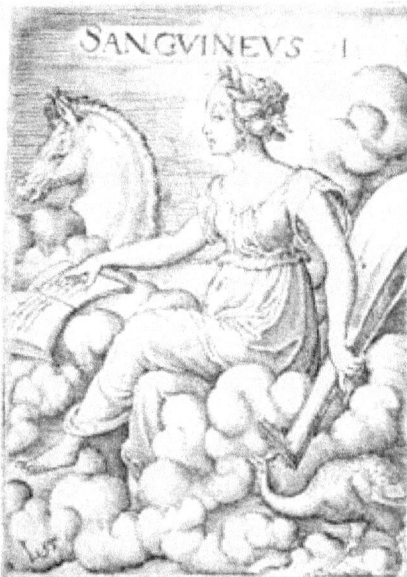

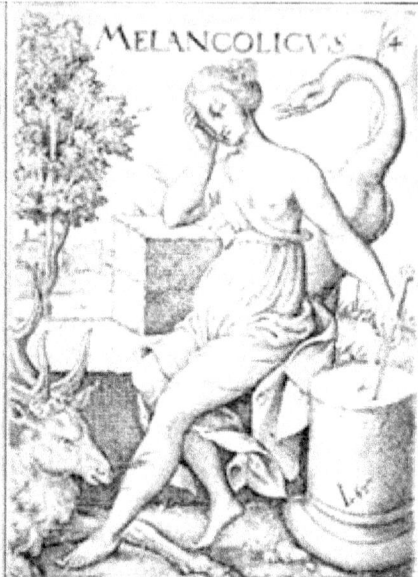

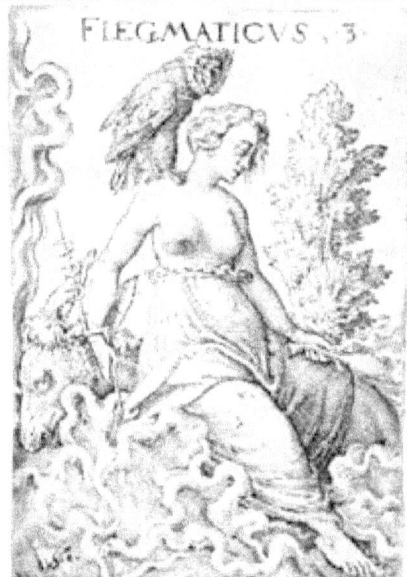

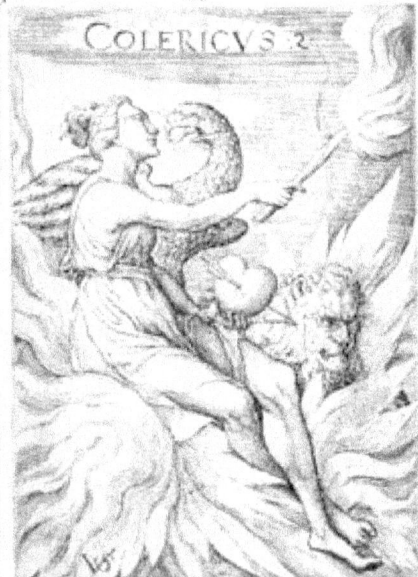

PART I - PRE 18th CENTURY HISTORY

I

Ancient roots of 18th century medicine

As incredible as it must seem today, when medicine progresses at such a speed as to make recent developments soon obsolete, much of the learning of 18th century physicians was based upon ancient writings, particularly those of Hippocrates (c450-c370 BC) and Galen (129-c200 AD). Not only was what they wrote concerning diagnosis, prognosis and treatment important for the practice of medicine during later times, their ideas about the cause of disease could still be found at the end of the 19th century.

The Hippocratic Legacy

According to all appearance the cause of disease should be found in the air, when it enters the body in excess, or in insufficient quantity, or too much at a time or when tainted by morbid miasmas. (Hippocrates)

While some aspects of the life of Hippocrates are known, for example, where he was born (the island of Cos near the western coast of what today is Turkey), the name of his father (Heraclides), and that he traveled widely practicing and teaching his medical arts, there is no certainty concerning what he wrote himself, since no writings have come directly from his time. Only after his death were writings associated with him compiled. These have come to be known as the *Hippocratic Corpus*, even though not all of the seventy texts included in the Corpus are written in the same style, nor are they without occasional contradictions. So much of importance is covered that Hippocrates has come to be known as the "Father of Medicine."

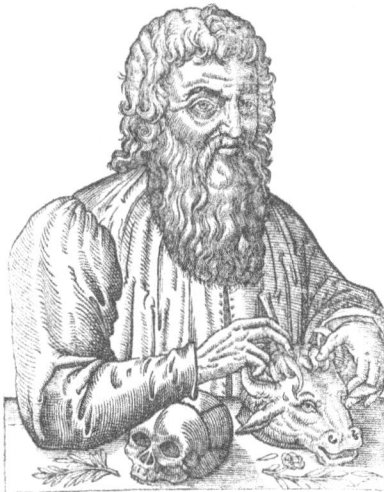

A key characteristic of the Hippocratic approach to medicine is the careful observation made of the history of individual sickness. Through these observations, Hippocratic physicians came to see illness as an orderly sequence of events involving body temperature, color of the skin, appearance of the eyes, prominence of the veins, pattern of breathing and the pulse, condition of the tongue, quality of the urine and feces, body position, and many other factors. These were recorded and those instances of particular interest were written up in the form of a case history to be used in the training of physicians. The language used to present clinical histories introduced medical terms that still are in active use - *acute, chronic, exacerbation, relapse, return, intermission, resolution, acme, paroxysm, crisis, protracted crisis,* and *convalescence,* to name just a few.

Much knowledge was gained of the natural course of illness. Great stress was placed on prognosis and the possibility of cure or of death of the patient. The ability to foretell outcomes of what before had been seen as events dictated by the gods no doubt contributed to public confidence in Hippocrates and his colleagues.

Disease was understood as a condition whereby the body no longer functioned well. The immediate cause of dysfunction was thought to be an imbalance of the body's 'humors' - the blood, yellow bile, black bile and phlegm. Humoral excess that brought on illness had to be driven out of the body. The body on its own would attempt this by using its *innate heat,* a heat that was thought to be generated in the heart and from which humors were created using food that had been eaten. The process whereby innate heat drove out excess humor was called *pepsis,* or *coction.* It resulted in the production of phlegm, pus, diarrhea, intestinal bleeding, nasal discharges and coughed-up mucus. If successful, the morbid material was adequately discharged and the patient recovered, otherwise not.

The Hippocratic physician was taught to direct his entire treatment to assist the innate healing power of the body and to avoid whatever might possibly antagonize it. An appropriate diet might be prescribed, possibly with some drugs. On occasion the knife would be used to open an abscess to help the body drive out the pus, thereby shortening the healing process.

The blood was thought to originate in the heart, yellow bile in the liver, black bile in the spleen, and phlegm in the brain. Each of these humors was associated with one of the four basic 'elements' from which the universe was built - air, fire, earth, and water. The humors with their associated substances were in turn linked to the four elementary properties (qualities) of hot, dry, cold and moist by a process of pairing:

blood (air) - moist and hot

yellow bile (fire) - hot and dry

black bile (earth) - dry and cold

phlegm (water) - cold and moist

The pairing of qualities allowed for the characterization of change in terms of one quality giving way to another. Secondary qualities could also be called upon, such as rare, dense, heavy, light, hard, soft and the like. This manner of conceiving matter had been refined by Aristotle and would dominate thinking until the 17th century when the atomic nature of matter came to the fore.

Humoral logic placed in evidence the role of the seasons. Phlegm (the cold-moist humor) increased in the winter. The moist and hot Greek spring was associated with an increase in blood, and the hot and dry summer with yellow bile. Finally, the cold, dry autumn brought on black bile. Nosebleeds, dysentery, bilious vomiting, catarrh, jaundice and various fevers - all could be related to one or more of the humors and seasons in which each humor predominated.

In his *Of the Epidemics,* Hippocrates described various "(epidemic) constitutions," which differed according to a range of meteorological factors, in particular, the nature and abundance of the rains, the direction of the dominating winds, and the seasonal timing of both the rains and the winds. To each constitution was ascribed particular illnesses. For example, a *"northerly state"* followed by *"droughts early in the spring"* and then a season *"inclined to the southerly,"* would yield *"ardent fevers ... in a few instances, and these very mild, being rarely attended with hemorrhage, and never proving fatal."* A wet, northerly winter followed by a cold spring, and a not too sultry summer, brought on *"dysenteric affections ... bilious diarrhea ... vomitings of bile, phlegm, and undigested food ..."* As reflected in the opening quote above, taken from *On Winds,* the pathological state of the atmosphere was ascribed to *"miasmas,"* whose original meaning in Greek is 'stain'.

The following text is a typical example of a Hippocratic statement concerning the importance of seasons. It is taken from the treatise *On Airs, Waters, and Places*:

Plague Legends

> *By respecting the seasons, one may judge whether the year will prove sickly or healthy from the following observations: - If the appearances connected with the rising and setting stars be as they should be; if there be rains in autumn; if the winter be mild; neither very tepid nor unseasonably cold, and if in spring the rains be seasonable, and so also in summer, the year is likely to be healthy. But if the winter be dry and northerly, and the spring showery and southerly, the summer will necessarily be of a febrile character, and give rise to ophthalmies and dysenteries ... for it is impossible, after such a spring, but that the body and its flesh must be loaded with humors, so that very acute fevers will attack all, but especially those of a phlegmatic constitution.*

From the many descriptions that appear in the different texts associated with the time of Hippocrates, medical experts have decided that smallpox, bubonic plague and measles were absent then, while malaria, diphtheria, and tuberculosis were very much present. The evidence for influenza and typhoid fever seems to be less certain.

Malarial fevers occupy a central place in the Corpus, so much so, that Paul F Russell (1894-1993), one of the great malariologists of the mid 20th century, argued that Hippocrates could also have been called the *"first malariologist."* No one before Hippocrates had so clearly and fully described the intermittent fevers that characterize the presence of malaria. The phenomenon of relapses is recognizable from his descriptions as well.

Malaria's seasonal and topographical variations were made evident along with its association with marshes. It was believed that those who drank stagnant marsh water would always have *"large, stiff spleens and hard, thin, hot stomachs, while their shoulders, collar bones and faces are emaciated (due to) the fact that their flesh dissolves to feed their spleens."* The prominence of the spleen in malaria no doubt explains its importance in the four-humor theory since the normal spleen is rather inconspicuous.

One of the more intriguing aspects of the Hippocratic Corpus is the lack of any reference to contagion as such. Several factors might help explain this important omission. First was the fact that the diseases whose contagiousness can most easily be recognized, i.e. smallpox and measles, were not present. Secondly was the presence of malaria. If malaria, with all of its periodic comings and goings, could be 'explained' by the prevailing epidemic constitution in conjunction with the theory of the four humors, there may not have been any other types of epidemic outbreak that could not be similarly explained. Still, it is to be noted that Hippocrates ignored the Great Plague of Athens about which Thucydides noted the *"rapidity with which men caught the infection; dying like sheep if they attended on one another."*

Rather than conjecture further on what can or cannot be found in the Hippocratic Corpus, we move on quickly to Galen, since his writings incorporated and built upon those of Hippocrates and served as basic texts for the medical community in the centuries that followed.

The Galenic Legacy

Even if we grant that this work (On the Nature of Man) was not by Hippocrates ... the idea that our bodies are generated and composed of these things (hot and cold and dry and wet) is Hippocratic doctrine. For in the most well known books of his, he seems to assume these origins, not only in considering the differences of diseases, but also thereafter in discovering the methods of curing. For diseases differ from each other with respect to hot and cold, wet and dry, and the treatment is to chill what is hot, and dry out what is wet; similarly, to heat what is cold and make wet what is dry. (Galen)

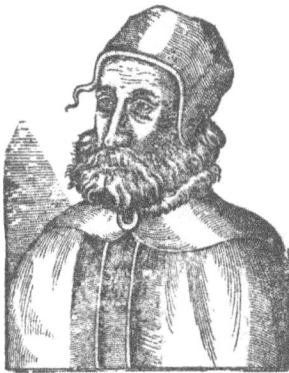

LIBER XXVI.
GALENI SECVNDVM HIPPOCRAD M MELCORVM PRÆSTANTISSIMI
Effigies.

Æ Quum erat Hippocratem diuino è femine, Diuum
Orbem muneribus conciliare sibi:
Scripta sed inuoluit tam multo ænigmate, verum
Vt quamuis solers nullus habere queat,
Pergamei auxilio nisi sint monimenta Galeni,
Qui docta ambages sustulit arte senis.
Ergo macte esto virtute arcana resoluens,

Galen was born in 130 AD at Pergamum in Mysia, Asia Minor (now Turkey). Pergamum was a center of learning with a library that afforded Galen opportunity for the study of medicine as well as philosophy and mathematics. There he had access to writings of earlier physicians. He used and judged these, drawing from them what suited best his way of thinking, to which he added his own results.

The work of Hippocrates occupied a central place in Galen's philosophy. He reviewed all of the commentaries on the Hippocratic Corpus, deciding for himself what was genuine and using it to build his own legacy. Most importantly, he helped create out of the diversity of the Corpus a coherent view, especially concerning the four 'classical' humors, and an allopathic principle of therapy, as reflected in the quote above.

Galen was a prolific writer. It is said that he kept at least 20 scribes on his staff to record his every word. He left posterity with voluminous tracts on all aspects of medicine, numbering around 500 books and treatises. His legacy was so great that opposing voices did not appear until the 16th century, and much of later thinking still was linked with that of Galen.

Galen, like other physicians of his time, employed philosophy to defend his medical theories and fight those who opposed Hippocrates. He did so in the best tradition of a trial lawyer. With Hippocrates and sometimes Aristotle on his side, he took on opposing schools by attacking important medical figures of the past with whom these schools were associated. One such school was that of the *Methodists,* which Galen associated with Asclepiades (c120-30 BC); this school criticized followers of Hippocrates as ones who, by observing and assisting nature - *"Meditated upon Death."*

A basic philosophical question that preoccupied Galen was what had changed in a person healthy one day and sick the next. This question was directly linked with what the body was composed of. Opposing the view that change involved the four humors were those who invoked atoms or other types of elements invisible to the naked eye. According to Asclepiades, for example, the human body was built of atoms, which joined to form its structural parts. Atoms were able to move through pores or canals, and health depended on this movement being free and without congestion. Disease resulted from a clogging of the pores and a stagnation of the atoms. It was particularly important that the atoms of the intestine circulate actively.

Followers of Asclepiades assumed that all solid parts of the body had the faculty of contracting or relaxing and that disease arose from abnormal contraction or relaxation in some part of the body. This theory led to simple methods of treatment, thus accounting for their name *Methodists.* The application of these methods were independent of any underlying theory of causation; they even believed that it was useless to consider the causes of disease, or even the organs affected by disease.

In one treatise after another Galen defended the four humors while attacking any atomistic or small-particle view of the body. In *Galen on the Elements According to Hippocrates* the argument is reduced to the absurd proposition that if the body was only composed on one element (atoms), all differential qualities of life would be impossible, e.g. - "*if man were one single thing, he would never suffer.*" Or, "*if they did suffer, they would suffer in one way only, so that there would be a single cure. But if this were true, clearly all medicine would be destroyed.*" Having decided that more than one element is needed, Galen goes on to explore the nature of such elements. After a long and to my mind somewhat tedious but no less intriguing exercise in logic, he arrives at the four elements that are at the foundation of the four-humor theory of Hippocrates:

> *And so you come again to fire and air and water and earth. In these alone will you find the qualities unmixed and unblended; the utmost heat and dryness in fire, the utmost coldness and wetness in water, and in each of the others according to their particular natures. And if you did not want to say that there are four elements, but rather two of them, or three, you will quickly have plenty of figuring to do.*

A similar kind of argumentation is then used to defend the proposition that the body is composed of four humors. These humors are "*another kind of element which is neither primary nor common, but particular to creatures with blood.*" All parts of the body are composed material but each is composed in its own way, thus, "*flesh, possessing blood, is soft and hot … sinew, being bloodless, is hard and cold.*" Blood, itself, is a composed matter. If the fibers carried in blood are removed, the blood no longer coagulates, and "*it differs in both color and composition.*" *Sometimes there is "an abundance of something thick and black in it … and sometimes it is red or white … indeed if you should cut open the veins of men who are still healthy -- out of one man the blood will flow yellow, out of another, red; out of another, whiter; and another, blacker.*" At which point Galen reminds his readers - "*if you wish to give the body a cathartic medicine, it will drain that humor which is suited by nature to draw out, but not equally in every nature of the body neither of healthy nor of sick men.*"

Almost immediately following this text, which is an excellent example of how Galen interweaves his natural with his therapeutic philosophy, he launches another broadside against Asclepiades:

> *Asclepiades, who attempts to overturn logically the good points of the discipline by means of amazing corpuscles and ducts, tries to persuade us that each medicine does not draw out its corresponding material, but that it changes and turns and alters the corrupting material -- whatever sort has been drawn out -- into its own nature. Then he says that the benefit that ensues comes about not because of the cleansing out of the offending*

> *material, but because of the general principle of draining. Thus Asclepiades'*
> *account is shameless when compared with the evidence … For if you should*
> *try to give a medicine which draws phlegm to a bile-ish man, know well*
> *that it is with no small harm that you will test this teaching.*

In his *On Hippocrates On the Nature of Man,* from which the opening quote above is taken, Galen continues the development of his ideas, and the battle against his detractors. We learn that those who were educated and who read his piece concerning *The Elements* "commended" it, while "*some uneducated people, who were unable to disprove any of the explanations in it, although they tried, were choked with jealousy, and they supposed that it would be sufficient slander to say that this work on which I was commenting is not by Hippocrates.*" This work is a long harangue, which adds little except the critical connection between the humors and his therapeutic method as seen in the following:

> *Who does not know that ailments occur, when someone goes outside in the*
> *excessively strong winter storms, and when someone goes out in excessive*
> *heat? Who does not suffer when they are thirsty or when they are*
> *completely filled with liquid…? And inflammations, and all ailments and*
> *natural afflictions, sometimes arise from excessive wetness flowing into the*
> *body part, and sometimes from the humors being naturally hot, or cold.*
> *And indeed the cure for a body over-filled with wetness is accomplished by*
> *means of draining, and the cure for a body dried by nature is by the*
> *addition of wetness, just as the cure for one which has been heated is by*
> *chilling, and for one which has been chilled beyond what is appropriate, by*
> *means of heat. And all medicines are shown to be effective by means of*
> *heating or cooling or drying or making wet.*

Continuing in this manner, Galen transformed the Hippocratic theory of the four humors into an elaborate but rigid pharmacological system. The order (if not false security) to drug therapy that this brought about was one which survived well into the 19th century. Therapy depended upon the determination of how warm or how dry the affected part was and adjusting the remedy accordingly. Also, the deeper the affected part was thought to be, the stronger the remedy in order for it not to lose its power on the way.

In addition to his pharmacological work Galen made important contributions to anatomy. He gained first-hand knowledge of living anatomy while serving as responsible physician for gladiators in the early part of his career. Open wounds provided a rare opportunity to explore the inner workings of the human body, an opportunity denied physicians by decrees that prohibited the dissection of human bodies. Afterwards, and of much greater importance,

Galen learned from the dissection of animals of all kinds, both living and dead.

Galen's preferred subject for studying physiology and anatomy was the macaque monkey (Barbary ape). It resembled a human being in appearance but, being smaller, permitted studies to be completed before decomposition set in. From these studies, among many other accomplishments, Galen demonstrated the role of the diaphragm in respiration and proved that the arteries contained blood. Previously it was believed that arteries, carrying only air, served as the conduits for the *pneuma*, the undefined and non-described 'spirit' that served to give life to humans. However, Galen did not recognize the circular nature of blood flow in the body. Instead, he imagined the heart functioning as a sponge that rhythmically soaked up the blood and squeezed it back into the body.

Galen presented his anatomical findings in his *On the Natural Faculties*. A similar pattern of presentation prevails, i.e. incorporation of Hippocrates' humors, judicious use of his own findings, and sarcastic assault on the ideas of his critics. His discussion of the kidneys illustrates all of these features.

It is common knowledge to all butchers that each kidney is attached to the bladder by a duct. Many people who suffer retention of urine feel pain in the regions between the kidney and the bladder. Both the retention and the pain cease upon passing of a stone. The obvious conclusion to draw is that the stone has passed through the connecting ducts, allowing the urine to flow unimpeded. But Asclepiades, who Galen supposes may never have seen "*a stone which had been passed by one of those sufferers,*" and about whom Galen is "*forced to marvel at the ingenuity of a man who puts aside these broad, visible routes,*" instead postulates "*others which are narrow, invisible - indeed, entirely imperceptible.*" Asclepiades imagines that what we drink turns into vapors which are absorbed into the bladder (sponge-like action) where they condense into urine. At that time the commonly held view was that the urine was produced in the bladder. Galen amuses himself for several paragraphs by imagining all of the other places in the body that these vapors might just as well have passed through or condensed into urine. He then describes several of his animal experiments in which he brilliantly demonstrated that in fact the urine originates in the kidneys and passes to the bladder through the ureter.

The function of the kidneys and the bladder demonstrates the "*forethought and art shown by nature*" and so praised by Hippocrates. Through the attraction of what is appropriate and the elimination of what is foreign, nature "*nourishes *the animal, makes it grow, and expels its disease by crisis."* There is in our bodies *"a concordance in the movements of air and fluid, and that everything is in sympathy."* According to Asclepiades, however, - *"nothing is naturally in sympathy with anything else, all substance being divided and broken up into inharmonious elements and absurd 'molecules'."*

Galen has been criticized for stifling medical progress. While it may seem exaggerated to blame him for what others did not do after his death, there is a sense in which this criticism seems justified. Galen placed himself as heir to the tradition of Hippocrates and Aristotle. As illustrated above, he denigrated all opposing schools of thought by mockery and insult. Instead of simply relying on his extensive accomplishments, most clearly evident in his experimental curative and anatomical work, he set his findings within a largely abstract philosophical debate with his opponents, a debate that invited others not to build on his science but to be entertained by the brilliancy of his argumentation and lulled into a false sense of security that his was the last word in medicine.

Galen had relatively little to say concerning the spread of diseases and possible causative factors. When he did write about such matters, he stuck very close to Hippocrates. Thus the unusual appearance of a disease which attacks many people (pestilence) arises from *"a modification of the air such that the seasons of the year do not preserve their proper order."* Plague (which covered for him more than bubonic plague) was brought about by a *"disastrous change in the character of the air making it prone to corruption."* where it is drawn in *"through the mouth like a poison."* He saw putridity of humors as the cause of acute fevers, favored by filthy living conditions. The initial cause of putridity was *"either a multitude of dead bodies which have not been burned or an exhalation from swamps or stagnant waters in the summer time."*

Galen recognized that certain diseases were contagious, as indicated by his warning that *"it is dangerous to associate with those who are afflicted of ophthalmia, skin diseases (scabies in Latin), phthisis and plague."* Nevertheless, the body must be predisposed for illness to occur; otherwise all would fall ill when the disease was present. On a very few occasions, one of which is quoted in Chapter III, Galen wrote of 'seeds' of disease. However, this occupied so minor a position in his writings in comparison to arguments paralleling the "epidemic constitution" of Hippocrates, that it would seem either that he did not believe in them, or that he could not mount a supportive argument worthy of his litigious talents!

Ancient Medicine Shaped by Christianity

There can be no question that the most magnificent service of all, one that is very necessary, one that is most sought by humanity, is the work that gives mankind a healthy mind in a healthy body. And even we can be good at this, if we join medicine to the priesthood. But because medicine without the favor of the heavens (as Hippocrates and Galen confessed, and as we have discovered, too) is very often worthless, in fact, very often harmful, it is no wonder that Astronomy belongs to this same charity of the priest's to which we said medicine also belongs. This kind of doctor, in my opinion, the sacred books compel us to honor, because the Almighty, out of necessity, created him. (Ficino)

It took six centuries before the Graeco-Roman pagan culture was transformed into a Christian one. Since, strictly speaking, Hippocrates, Plato, Aristotle and Galen were all pagans, one outcome of this transition could have been the total rejection of Hippocratic medicine. This did not happen. Instead, Christian medicine adapted ancient medicine to suit its spiritual as well as bodily needs, and in so doing, moved the center of gravity of medical practice from the bedside to somewhere intermediate between the patient and the heavens, as witness Marsilio Ficino's invocation above. Ficino (1433-1499) was a 15th century Italian philosopher, philologist, physician and ordained priest. His translations of ancient texts had a great influence on medical beliefs and practices as discussed in Chapter III.

Hippocratic medicine, i.e. all ancient medicine that drew its inspiration from the Hippocratic tradition, was well established by the 1st century AD. As described earlier, Galen was successful in rejecting competing schools and establishing his interpretation of the Hippocratic Corpus as the dominant school of medicine. The Hippocratic tradition particularly thrived in the East where it was taken up by Arab scholars in the 9th century, refined and reintroduced back into Europe during the centuries that followed. In the Christian areas of Europe, however, this tradition came under severe questioning. Particularly suspect was the ancient medical tradition that placed great importance on the health of the soul; Hippocratic physicians were encouraged to treat both the body and the soul. For Christians, however, the soul was God's domain. Secular physicians had no business with it; only the Church could address its 'ills'.

Galen doubted the immortality of the soul, thus taking a position contrary to that of Plato who, in several of his works, claimed not only that the individual soul survived death but that it existed before birth as part of a Universal Soul. This did not prevent Galen, however, from indicating that anyone pursuing *"the art of hygiene"* must *"shape the health of the soul"* as well, *"lest it (the body) slip into disease."* The soul's importance lay in its association with many of the key organs of the body, i.e. the heart, brain, and liver. Plato had located the immortal soul in the part nearest heaven, the head, while Galen envisaged the mortal soul to be distributed between the heart and the liver. Aristotle accepted these three souls, although he ascribed somewhat different purposes to each than Plato had; also, he firmly re-established the heart as the seat of the soul. The belief in multiple souls was totally unacceptable to Christian dogma.

The Christian soul was immortal but not divine and co-eternal with God, as Plotinus (205-270AD), the greatest of the Neo-Platonists philosophers, had proposed. The Platonic soul was devoid of corruption and sin and thus had no need of redemption, a position equally antagonistic to Christian thought. Augustine (354-430AD) argued that the soul was neither part of God nor the body, but was absolutely and continuously dependent on God for its existence and continuance in being. Sin and all moral evil, according to Augustine, derived from the soul turning away from eternal Truth and Good towards the temporal and material, as lived by the corporeal body.

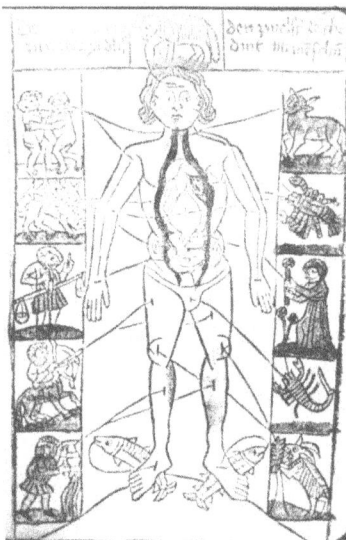

In addition to God, souls and bodies, the universe also contained celestial bodies, where pagans placed their gods. Particularly important was the Upper Cosmos above the moon. As depicted by Ptolemy (*fl.*140AD), and not challenged until Nicolas Copernicus (1473-1543), the earth stood in the center of a universe around which the moon, sun and planets moved in circular orbits; the stars were fixed on the outer-most shell, which Aristotle had determined to be the 55th one removed from the earth. Christians reacted strongly against all religious connotations that Plotinus and other pagan philosophers had ascribed the cosmos; all veneration of heavenly bodies was rejected. But not rejected was the possibility that the planets, stars, moon and sun could influence the human condition, including health.

Astrology lay outside the Hippocratic-Galenic tradition. The brief reference to the Dog-star and Arcturus in Hippocrates' *Of the Epidemics* refers to the time of year not to any astral influence. Also not included in the Hippocratic Corpus was the possibility that the gods could influence the health of individuals. Hippocrates conceived sickness as a natural process born of natural causes. Even epilepsy, the so-called divine disease, he argued was "*no more divine or more sacred than other diseases, but has a natural cause ... its supposed divine origin is due to men's inexperience.*" This position was a dramatic break with earlier practice that invoked divine causes and sought treatment by means of repentance of sins committed, expiatory rituals, expulsion of demons, or making offering to the gods. This was a break that did not survive the arrival of Christianity, which, like earlier Judaism, accepted that God could punish sinners with disease as well as use disease to test the faith of the righteous. The extra-terrestrial nature of disease gave credence to astrological interpretations of disease causation, a practice that blossomed following the great astronomical advances made by Islamic science.

Evil spirits, as well, found their way into the Christian cosmology with the New Testament providing example after example of how disease was caused by demons. Exorcism was needed to cast out the devil and heal the sick. Augustine categorically claimed that "*all diseases are to be ascribed to demons.*"

God inflicting illness upon mankind opened up the possibility that faith could bring about cures of what otherwise would seem to be certain death or chronic disability. Miraculous cures did not cease with the death of Jesus, as attested by Augustine who reported on 25 miracles that were wrought in his lifetime alone. It was also Augustine who preached strongly that "*from its beginning all the progeny of mankind was damned ... from the body itself arise so many diseases that not even the books of the doctors contain them all.*" Individuals could be saved from original sin, but only through faith and belief in a Christian God. The belief that Christianity offered a powerful weapon against disease was certainly one of the more attractive features of this new religion.

Miracles were understood to be the works of the saints; diseases were assigned to the special care of particular saints. Thus, for example, St Anthony was called upon for erysipelas (St Anthony's fire), St Blaise for goiter, St Christopher for epilepsy, St Roch for plague boboes, and St Sebastian for pestilence. Many healing shrines established during the middle ages continue to this day.

Thus by the time of 15th century, when Ficino lived, disease had become deeply embedded in the Christian culture, with God, angels, demons and saints seen as playing major roles both in their origin as well as their cure. Christian medicine gave a role to the supernatural that Hippocratic medicine had not. One consequence was that medicine was led away from a systematic investigation of nature, a direction even the dogmatic Galen had argued for. Christian belief in the supernatural allowed, at least as expressed by Ficino and other Christian Neo-Platonists, a place for magic. More importantly, as already noted, Ficino's translations of Neo-Platonic and other ancient writings made more credible the long and well-established tradition of superstition, charms and incantations, along with other occult and magical forms. How these beliefs affected thinking concerning the origin of epidemic disease is explored further in Chapter III.

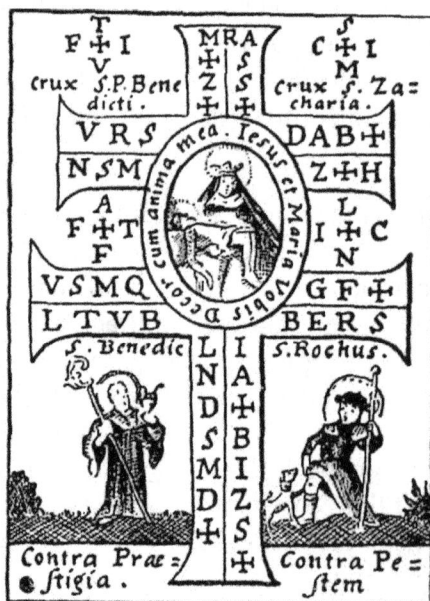

II

Decline of Galenism and the Rise of New Schools of Medicine

The Black Death of the 14th century shattered medieval institutions and left in its wake a vacuum from which arose the Renaissance. Starting in Italy, in mid-14th century, the Renaissance saw a dramatic revival of interest in the classic writings of ancient Greece and Rome. This return to the past was part of a wider Humanistic movement that celebrated poetry, eloquence, painting, architecture, sculpture, music and singing, and studied the relationship between the material and spiritual world, especially as shaped by Neo-Platonic philosophies.

The 'rediscovery' of the classics of ancient Greece and Rome led to a great effort to find original manuscripts, including those of Hippocrates and Galen. A whole host of learned and able medical authors were involved. It was felt particularly important to uncover Galen's original Greek manuscripts in order to use them to remove the contaminating elements that had been added over more than one millennium. Furthermore, not all of Galen had been translated and some of his works were available only in an abridged form.

In 1500 there appeared the first printing of a genuine Galenic text in the original Greek. This was followed by the Aldine Press Galen in 1525, an extensive compilation of Galen's writings, also in the original Greek. The reaction to this publication was mixed, due to many errors that were introduced during its rapid production, but it did lead to a strengthening of Galen's hold on the teaching of medicine. For the first time in the 'modern' western world, all facets of Galen's work were presented anew. His *On my opinions of Hippocrates and Plato* demonstrated his synthesis of ancient philosophy and medicine. His anatomical investigations were made clear in detail, and practical therapy gained as well from new material concerning bloodletting and drug use.

Ironically, with the Humanists also came the Reformation, a revolt against the authority of the Church, which inspired a revolt against traditional authority in medicine, vested largely in the writings of Galen. It would appear that the drive to resurrect the 'original' Galen motivated the anti-Galenists to action. This revolt led to demonstrations of errors committed by Galen and the introduction of new therapeutic methods that went outside the traditional

Galenic approach. Nevertheless, the hold that Galen had on medical thinking was such that it would still be some time before the last remnants of his works would be eclipsed for good.

Many physicians questioned some aspect of the Galenic corpus. However, most questioned in silence to avoid attracting any attention to themselves during this religiously tumultuous era. From those that did contribute to the fall of Galenism, three particularly stand out in importance - Paracelsus (1493-1541) and Andreas Vesalius (1514-1564) in the 16th century and William Harvey (1578-1658) in the 17th century. Paracelsus and Vesalius expressed their opposition vociferously and widely, and both contributed something dramatically new to the practice of medicine - Paracelsus, in the domain of treatment - Vesalius, in anatomy.

Paracelsus wrote extensively, but much of his work was suppressed by the medical establishment and remained unpublished during his lifetime. Vesalius, relying on the advent of the printing press, published a large and attractive illustrated work on anatomy of great educational value. Harvey, on the other hand, with little fanfare and in one fell swoop, refuted the major Galenic error concerning the movement of the blood, and introduced a much more scientific approach to anatomical and physiological research than had existed before.

It is difficult to appreciate from such a long distance the dangers these and other natural philosophers, as they were called then, ran while pursuing their studies. For example, in 1553, Michael Servetus (1511-53), a Spanish theologian and physician who may have been the first to describe the blood circulation between the heart and the lungs, was put to the stake in Geneva, the home of Calvinism. His description was written into a tractate, the *Christianismi Restitutio*, considered heretical by the church. Only three copies of this publication survived his death. The other copies along with all of his other publications were added to the pyre of slow burning green wood to help fuel the fire that consumed his body. More than another hundred years would pass before Charles II of England in 1676 forced the removal of the death penalty for the crimes of atheism, blasphemy, heresy and other religious offences. Nevertheless, this did not prevent a medical student aged 18 named Aikenhead from being accused of heresy and hanged in 1696 in Edinburgh. The fact of the matter is that physicians were dealing with questions that were so intimately related to religious beliefs that they could not help but offend some sects with their ideas. Some, for example van

Helmont and Fludd, who we will meet later, seemed to deliberately seek confrontation with religious authorities, often at the risk of their lives.

Although the 17th century was still dominated by mystical attitudes and beliefs, the work of Harvey and others reflect a clear trend towards the application of scientific methods, e.g. clear descriptions of methods used, increased use of measurement in experimentation, and a growing number of investigators who sought to explain Nature in terms that did not rely upon occult properties.

The Revolt of Paracelsus

*I am directing you, physicians, to alchemy for the preparation of the **magnalia** (divine substance), for the production of the **mysteria**, for the preparation of the **arcana** (a powerful secret remedy), for the separation of the pure from the impure, to the end that you may obtain a flawless, pure remedy, God-given, perfect, and of certain efficacy, achieving the highest degree of virtue and power. (Paracelsus)*

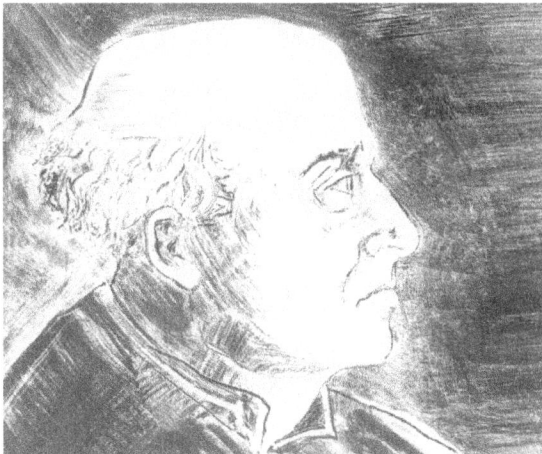

The revolt against the established traditions of Galenic medicine, that was smoldering in the early part of the 16th century, culminated in a personality of unique and striking character who went by the name of Paracelsus (1493-1541). His real name was Philippus Theophrastus Aureolus Bombastus von Hohenhiem.

Paracelsus was born in Switzerland in 1493. His father, a physician in a mining town in Austria, taught him the rudiments of botany, chemistry, metallurgy and medicine while Paracelsus was still quite young. At that time, mineralogy and metallurgy were advanced in the application of the methods of technical chemistry, including quantitative ones. Having acquired a working knowledge of chemistry and medicine early in his life, Paracelsus was not your normal student of medicine when he attended the University of Ferrara in Italy around the age of twenty. He had learned from his father that nothing of value was to be found in the ancient texts of Galen or the more recent ones from Arabic medicine. He quickly joined other scholars who were questioning the validity of these ancient medical texts. Exceptionally, Paracelsus had only enthusiastic praise to offer for the work of Ficino, characterizing him as a *"great physician."*

Paracelsus lived a turbulent life in turbulent times. He was quarrelsome and rebellious. He was often drunk and poorly dressed, and his manner of speech was 'bombastic' leading some later to erroneously consider his a mocking nickname. Legend has it that his irritable nature was due to his having been emasculated by a drunken soldier when he was a youth. Other legends ascribe this condition to an encounter with a wild boar. He, himself, suggested the influence of his early environment:

> *I know I am not the kind that speaks to each only that which might please him; I am not used to giving submissive answers to arrogant questions. I know my ways, and I do not wish to change them; neither could I change my nature. I am a rough man, born in a rough country. I have been brought up among pines, and I may have inherited some knots.*

Rather than completing his studies in Italy Paracelsus chose to seek knowledge his own way, a search that took him far and wide. Sometimes fleeing his enemies, other times moving on in search of newer adventures, his travels took him all over Europe, including the British Isles and possibly the Near East. He was employed as a military surgeon in a number of mercenary armies, and on different occasions served as court physician to royal families. Through travel, Paracelsus came to *"recognize many various diseases … and many things."* For, as he said - *"He who would explore nature must tread her books with his feet."*

For a short period of time he taught medicine at Basle, but this ended when his influential local supporter died. While at Basle, Paracelsus refused to teach in Latin and instead used the local vernacular German of Switzerland (Schweizerdeutsch), in which all of his writings are written. He showed some respect for Hippocrates but spoke contemptuously of Galen, who he claimed was *"in hell"* and less learned than *"his shoe buckles."*[1] Perhaps, owing to his

---

[1] According to Dante both Galen and Hippocrates were in 'limbo' because they were pagans. On the other hand, he condemned Epicure and his followers to circle VI of hell because they believed that the soul dies when the body dies. This suggests that Dante was

deep Christian faith, Paracelsus could forgive Hippocrates but not Galen who doubted the immortality of the soul, a belief not associated with Hippocrates.

Following one of his 'inspirational' lectures, his students burned the works of Galen in the market place along with those of the renowned Arabic physician Avicenna (980-1037). Paracelsus' assault on the ancients was no less violent than that of Luther against the Pope. Not without reason was he called the 'Luther of medicine.' Following Luther, he abandoned Latin and wrote extensively in his own language; it is his writings that inspired many of his readers to follow in his footsteps.

True medicine, Paracelsus asserted, rested upon four pillars—philosophy, the virtue of the physician, astronomy and alchemy. Philosophy embraced all the sciences and was not limited to Aristotle for whom he had little use. Virtue was a necessary prerequisite to be a good physician. Instead of virtuous physicians, Paracelsus saw only avarice and ignorance among his medical colleagues. Provoked to a frenzy of invective against his profession, Paracelsus was 'rewarded', not only by their vocal opposition but, as well, by strong censure of his writings and beliefs. So effective was the boycott of his ideas that only a few of his writings were published during his lifetime, as noted earlier.

As we will explore in the next chapter, much of what Paracelsus had to say reflected the then-prevalent ideas concerning the applicability of astrology to medicine. Even Paracelsus' ideas concerning alchemy derived from a relatively long tradition. But Paracelsus broke important new grounds concerning therapeutical practice, grounds that revolutionized the use of drugs for treatment.

In his treatise *On the Miner's Sickness*, Paracelsus introduced one of the most basic features of his alchemical belief, namely the substance of sulfur, mercury and salt:

> *Know then concerning the lung-sickness that it comes through the power of the stars, in that their peculiar characters are boiled out, settling on the lungs in three different ways: in a mercurial manner like the sublimated smoke that coagulates, like a salt spirit which passes from resolution to*

---

probably not as versed as Paracelsus was concerning the beliefs of Galen. In any case, it is not likely that Paracelsus relied on Dante at all since alchemists are assigned to a much deeper level in Dante's hell!

> *coagulation, and thirdly, like a sulfur which is precipitated on the walls by roasting.*

Sulfur represents the gaseous in matter which burns, mercury the fluid in matter which evaporates when heated, and salt the solid in matter which resists heat. Paracelsus believed that the four elements of fire, water, air and earth, from which the world is made, are **only** composed of these three substances - *"For they form everything that lies in the four elements, they bear in them all the forces and faculties of perishable things."*

Syphilis, a disease that first appeared in Europe following the voyage of Columbus to the New World, occupied much of Paracelsus' time and energy. In his pamphlet, an *Essay on the French Disease,* subtitled, *About Impostors,* Paracelsus took the whole medical faculty and guild to task for the use of guaiac as well as for their indiscriminate and clumsy use of mercury, the other approach then in vogue for treating syphilis:

> *This patient you have smoked fifteen times. That one you have balmed fifteen times. Another you have washed fifteen times. And the fourth you led around in the (guaiac) wood. This one you made swallow a quarter pound of mercury, another half a pound or a pound or even a pound and a half. This one has it in his marrow, another in his veins. There is it in a corpse; there in a living man goes around with it. There it is in powdered form; there it is sublimated, calcinated, resolved, precipitated, and so on. Who could cover up such a felony?*

Paracelsus' great book on syphilis contains some of the best clinical descriptions of the disease available at that time. For treatment he advocated sulfur baths and mercury balms in much diluted form, thus sparing his patients purgation, salivation, hunger and sweat cures. Whereas other physicians applied mercury in an indiscriminate manner, Paracelsus applied specific quantities of a particular compound. Finding the correct dosage of any given chemical was critical in his approach to treatment:

> *You rebuke me for my prescriptions: consider yours, how they are. First, for instance, with your purging. Where in all your books is a Purgatio that is not poison, or serves not death, or can be used without annoyance, if Dosis is not given in proper weight?*

Paracelsus explained life, health and disease in terms of the three substances, sulfur, mercury and salt. Although he occasionally acknowledged some role for the traditional four humors, it was always of secondary importance. He envisaged much of organic disease in terms of excess sulfur, mercury or salt.

For example, gout was seen as being caused by a crystal deposit of *tartar* in the joints. Galenic physicians had argued that aging caused it and hence it was incurable. Paracelsus claimed, with apparently some success in his practice, that these crystals could be dissolved by potassium tartrate.

Alchemy, as expressed in the opening quote above, was to be used by physicians to separate the 'evil' from the 'good' in their common cause. Paracelsus justified this approach by arguing that it is far easier to seek an *arcanum* (powerful secret remedy) that works for everyone than it is to seek an individual cure for each instance of a specific disease:

> *If the specialist wants to seek a special diet and a special prescription for each one (many kinds of jaundice), he will seek too long to be able to help the patient.*

Although it has been argued by some that Paracelsus' view of disease was similar to that of later centuries, his impact was almost exclusively in the field of chemistry, a word that he may have been the first to use. He rejected the dominant polypharmacy in favor of simple medicaments - *"It is better to know and to understand one remedy ... nature does not call for long recipes."* He introduced several new drugs or drugs little used in the past, including mercury, lead, sulfur, iron, arsenic and copper sulfate. He had a great preference for the alcoholic extracts (tinctures), including laudanum (an opiate based tincture). Many of these remedies had been in use before, but Paracelsus and his followers placed their study at the forefront of medicine. Pharmacy was thereby enriched, not only through the introduction of a number of chemicals for therapy, but also by his endeavor to extract the *"healing virtue"* from the more or less inert substances in which he thought it would be hidden, their so-called *"quintessence."*

The impact of Paracelsus on medicine was not immediate. Controversy surrounded his name well after his death. Some of his remedies were quickly adopted but his pharmacological approach to dosage took a longer time before it was appreciated. Many of his followers were mystical quacks and impostors, but others, as discussed below, of better repute, brought to therapy a whole new outlook by the chemical procedures that they developed and by the chemical drugs that thus were created.

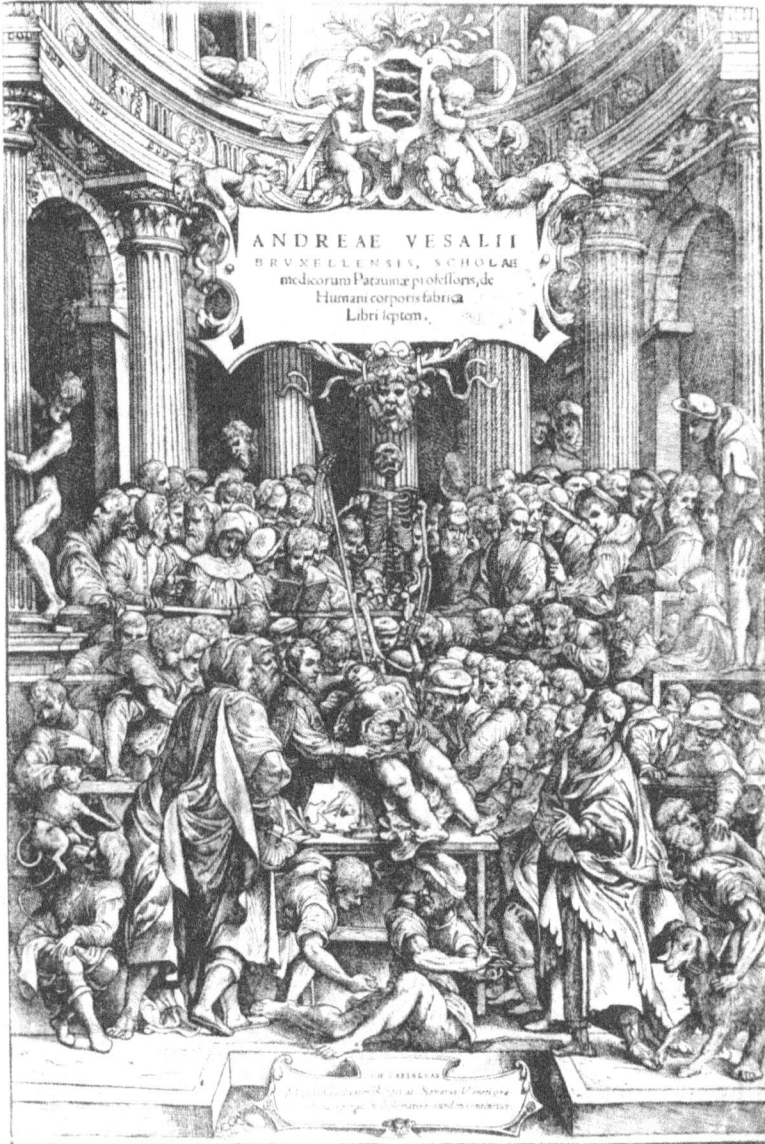

ANDREAE VESALII
BRVXELLENSIS, SCHOLAE
medicorum Patauinæ profefforis, de
Humani corporis fabrica
Libri feptem.

BASILEAE.

Galen's Anatomy Revisited by Vesalius

*The whole lot of them have placed their faith in him (Galen), with the result that you can not find a doctor who has thought that even the slightest slip has ever been detected in the anatomical volumes of Galen, much less **could** be found (now). (Vesalius)*

Vesalius, like Paracelsus, had a physician father, complained about how medicine was taught, and did much of his medical education in Italy. There, their similarity ends. Vesalius was attracted to the University of Padua, not by its strongly developed medical-astrological culture, but instead by the opportunity offered there to learn anatomy by dissection, knowledge that Paracelsus claimed to be of little use, and better left for *"Italian jugglers."*

Vesalius was born in Brussels in 1514 in a family that boasted three generations of doctors who had collected the finest ancient medical manuscripts. The house in which he was born and grew up was near the site where criminals were executed and their bodies left to rot. As a child he demonstrated a strong interest in anatomy; he dissected small field animals such as rats, moles, and dormice, along with occasional stray cats and dogs he came across.

His education was not untypical of many physicians at that time. From the University of Louvain, which he entered at the age of 15, he moved on to Paris in 1533 for his medical education. There he spent his first year studying Hippocrates, Galen and other writers of the past. His second year was devoted entirely to Galen's anatomy, about which, later, he would say that he learned virtually nothing. Not content with the rare opportunities afforded him at the University to do his own dissections, he obtained what body parts he could find by foraging cemeteries, seeking graves that had caved in, and visiting Montfaucon, the site in Paris where the bodies of criminals were brought to hang and disintegrate before being placed in a vault. Back in his room he would soak the parts in vinegar to disguise the terrible stench and then by candlelight dissect them until all hours in the morning.

Being forced to leave Paris when war broke out between France and the Holy Roman Empire in 1535, he first made his way to Louvain and then Brussels where his anatomical demonstrations were not well received. Local theologians did not at all appreciate his remarks on the location of the soul. Advised that Italian Universities would be more willing to welcome his revolutionary approach, he proceeded to Padua where he obtained his doctoral degree in 1537 and was appointed professor of surgery and anatomy on the day following his graduation! Padua, like other Italian schools of medicine, actively promoted the study of man's body including opening up the human body for anatomical demonstrations. A renewed interest in dissection was one of the more important consequences of Renaissance humanism.

From the first day as professor Vesalius taught anatomy in a totally revolutionary, 'hands on' manner. Traditionally, the professor of anatomy would sit in an elevated structure provided with steps and a reading desk, something like a pulpit. There, high above the body to be dissected, he would read from a classical text, most often that of Galen, while the actual dissection would be performed by individuals with little or no anatomical knowledge. The whole purpose of the exercise was not to learn anything new but to demonstrate that what Galen had written was correct. Vesalius opined that *"fewer facts are placed before the spectators in that tumult than a butcher could teach a doctor in his meat market."*

Vesalius did not start out with the idea of discrediting Galen. On the other hand, he was talented and ambitious and knew how to exploit the newly arrived power of the printing press. At the same time that he used each dissection to improve his understanding of human anatomy, he used each occasion to refine large charts to graphically illustrate his findings. Within 4 months he had accumulated enough material for the publication of six charts with accompanying text. Each chart was printed on woodcut plates 19 by 13½ inches in size. Although there were some non-conforming observations, these illustrations largely followed Galenic doctrine. They still showed, for example, the erroneous five lobed liver (of a dog), and the *rete mirabile* (to be found in an ape but not in humans).

The student body of Bologna invited Vesalius in 1540 to give a series of anatomical demonstrations. It is during this period that Vesalius came to realize that Galen's anatomy was not based on the human body but instead on different animals. He not only found many errors in Galen but also was able to show on which animals Galen had based his erroneous anatomy. On his return to Padua, he immersed himself in documenting carefully more than 200 inaccuracies, some of which were the key points in the Galenic corpus. He announced openly that Galen had been *"deceived by his monkeys."*

In 1543, at the age of 28, Vesalius published his masterpiece, *De Humani Corporis Fabrica* (On Man's Bodily Works). For this he chose the best artists available, the best printers and a distributor who quickly made it available throughout Europe. The full publication consisted of 663 folio pages, 11 large plates and almost 300 other illustrations.[2] In it he exhorted his readers to do their own dissection and provided instructions for that purpose. They were advised to *"begin to put faith in their own not ineffectual sight and powers of reason rather than in the writings of Galen."*

Vesalius dedicated his text to *"the Divine Charles the Fifth, Greatest and Most Invincible Emperor."* He did so seeking to protect himself from the onslaught of criticism that he knew had to follow his having demonstrated so many errors in Galen. His father had been a *"most faithful chief pharmacist"* for the Emperor and Vesalius had already had occasion to show his earlier works to Charles. All of this was to no avail. The Galenists attacked the publication. Even his students accused him of plagiarizing their ideas.

Vesalius made the mistake of asking Jacobus Sylvius (1478-1555), his anatomy teacher in Paris, an arch Galenist, what he thought of his work! Sylvius believed Galen to be *"infallible,"* claiming that any advance past Galen *"was impossible."* Not only did Sylvius publicly assault Vesalius, he proceeded to spend the next 8 years elaborating his response - *A Refutation of the Slanders of a Madman Against the Writings of Hippocrates and Galen.* In this 'work', Sylvius wrote - *"it would have been easier to cleanse the Augean stables than to remove even the worse lies from this hodgepodge made of thefts and bloated with slanders....,"* and implored his imperial Majesty *"to punish severely, as he deserves, this monster born and bred in his own house..."* Furthermore, like many of his contemporaries, Sylvius believed that illustrations contaminated anatomical texts.

Sylvius demanded that Vesalius retract his errors, to which Vesalius challenged him, in effect, to a 'duel' next to a cadaver where he would see with his own eyes *"where lies the truth."* Whether in response to the invective that his *Fabrica* had wrought, or for other reasons, six months after its

---

[2] Leonardo de Vinci produced outstanding anatomical drawings several decades before Vesalius but unfortunately he never realized his plan to produce and publish an anatomical treatise. Instead they remained as isolated fragments for centuries. However, the text that accompanied his illustrations mostly adhered to the traditional Galenic view of human anatomy, although for a while, de Vinci followed Aristotle in believing that the heart rather than the liver was the blood-making organ.

publication Vesalius burnt all of his notes and manuscripts, including his priceless annotation of Galen, and accepted an offer from Charles V to serve as physician at the imperial court. He was never to conduct anatomical research again, although it is believed that at the time of his accidental death in 1564 he was making his way back to Padua to take on a newly liberated and well endowed post of professor of anatomy.

Vesalius did not develop any intrinsic anatomical conception of disease. For that matter, there is no indication that de Vinci had either. However, while de Vinci adopted the doctrine of humors, giving the blood a prominent place in the maintenance of good health, Vesalius ascribed illness to *"affected portions"* of the body, indicating that cure depended on knowing those parts.

Harvey's Explorations of the Heart and Blood

When I first tried animal experimentation for the purpose of discovering the motions and functions of the heart by actual inspection and not by other people's books, I found it so truly difficult that I almost believed with Fracastoro that the motion of the heart was to be understood by God alone. (Harvey)

The heart played a central role in ancient physiology. It was imagined that the heart receives from the lungs the life-giving *pneuma*[3], which it then pumps through the arteries to all parts of the body. Until Galen proved that the arteries carried blood, it was believed that they were filled only with the pneuma. Also, it was thought that the rhythmic expansion and contraction of the pneuma contained in the arteries gave rise to the pulsation present in all living humans. The pulse was seen to be synchronous with the expansion of the heart, occurring when the heart struck the chest. This would correspond to the diastole, i.e. the moment when the heart was fully inflated.

Galen had elaborated a complex system to account for the flow of the blood and different pneuma thought to exist. Following previous thought, he believed that blood originated in the liver, but that it was generated as and when needed by the different parts of the body. In addition, the liver imbued blood with a particular pneuma innate in all living substance. This pneuma was known as the *natural spirit*. The natural spirit carrying blood entered the

---

[3] The pneuma was equivalent to both soul and life, and could be imagined to be 'seen' rising as a shimmering steam from the shed blood of sacrificial victims.

heart on its right side. There its impurities would be removed and sent to the lungs where they were exhaled. Once purified the blood would ebb back into the body through the venous system.

Galen also believed in a *vital spirit,* a pneuma that entered the body from the lungs (trachea and pulmonary vein). This pneuma was carried by the arterial system to the base of the brain where it was minutely divided by the channels of the *rete mirable* (a network of nerves and vessels at the base of the brain shown by Vesalius not to be present in humans). In that supposed human organ, the blood became charged with yet a third pneuma, the *animal spirit,* which was distributed by the nerves, which were thought to be hollow.

The movement of the *vital spirit* raised the question of how it found its way from the venous to the arterial system. For this purpose Galen imagined that there must exist pores in the septum that divide the right and left ventricles. Vesalius denied the existence of these pores; in fact, this was one of the key points that most upset the Galenists. However, Vesalius was not able to work out how blood circulated. This was left for William Harvey to accomplish.

Harvey was born in Folkestone, England in 1578. He came from a well-to-do family from which he derived total economic security. He learned Latin and Greek early and was well versed in the classics. He received his BA in 1597 and went to Padua for his medical studies. There, he came under the influence of the great anatomist Giralomo Fabrizio (c1533-1619) whose discovery of the valves in the veins would later prove vital to Harvey's own discoveries. He received his doctoral diploma in 1602 and returned to England.

Very little is actually known of Harvey's personal life since, unlike Galen and Vesalius, he did not include any autobiographical details in his scientific writings. Those writings seem to begin seriously in 1615 when he was appointed Lumleian Lecturer of the College of Physicians, a major post which required him to give two public lectures each week in a six-year cycle. Harvey accepted this responsibility until 1656, when he voluntarily gave up the office.

His lecture notes, found only in 1876, indicate that he began to consider the question of circulation of the blood long before the publication of his magnum opus in 1628 - *Exercitatio Anatomica de Motu Cordis et Sanquinis in Animalibus* - An Anatomical Essay on the Motion of the Heart and Blood in Animals - *De Motu Cordis,* for short. In the first part, which it is thought he worked out some ten years before the second, Harvey described the movement of the heart with its associated in- and out-flow of blood. In the second part he introduced the concept that the blood travels through the body in a never-ending circular cycle.

In order to study the heart's movement, which Harvey characterized as twitches *"coming and going like a flash of lightning,"* he made observations on a host of vivisected animals. Cold-blooded snakes, because of the slow beating of their hearts, were favored, as well as dogs and pigs just before their death when the heart motion slows and is easier to follow. From these studies he concluded that the heart contracts forcibly to drive its contained blood out into the major arteries at which time the arteries dilate. The pulse is synchronous with the heart's contraction or systole and is caused by it. During contraction, the heart's length increases and its apex strikes the chest wall. In between heartbeats, the heart is passively filled by blood flowing in from the periphery of the body by way of the veins. Harvey clearly described both heart-lung and heart-body blood flows.

In the second half of *De Motu Cordis*, Harvey introduced something new to physiological research - the use of measurement. Harvey was apparently aware of its novelty since he returns to it again and again in the course of his presentation. First he estimated that the capacity of the ventricle in the human heart, i.e. that part of the heart which contains the blood destined for the body following each contraction, to be around 2 to 3 ounces. From this figure he calculated that every hour the heart pumped some 540 pounds of blood into the aorta, i.e. some three times the average person's weight! Knowing where the blood entered the heart, the remaining question was from where? - the only logical answer was - the veins.

It was at this point that he benefited from Fabrizio's discovery that there were valves in the veins. Harvey demonstrated that these valves served the purpose of preventing the blood from flowing away from the heart, which clearly supported his conjecture that the role of the veins was to carry the returning blood to the heart. Harvey could not, however, describe what pathway was used for the blood to move from the arteries to the veins; he hypothesized the existence of what he called 'pores', at the same time lamenting *"Damn it, no such pores exist, nor can they be demonstrated!"* Harvey's pores, as opposed to those Galen believed to be present in the heart, would be shown to exist. This was in 1660, when Marcello Malpighi of Bologna demonstrated the existence of capillaries using a microscope.

There is perhaps some irony in the fact that Harvey has not been criticized for basing his theory of blood circulation in humans on results largely drawn from observations made on animals. This point, however, cannot be pushed too far. Harvey's experiments are described clearly; no effort is made to hide the nature of the animals under study. Galen, it would seem, chose to obscure matters, leaving readers to imagine that his results stemmed from studies involving observations made on human bodies.

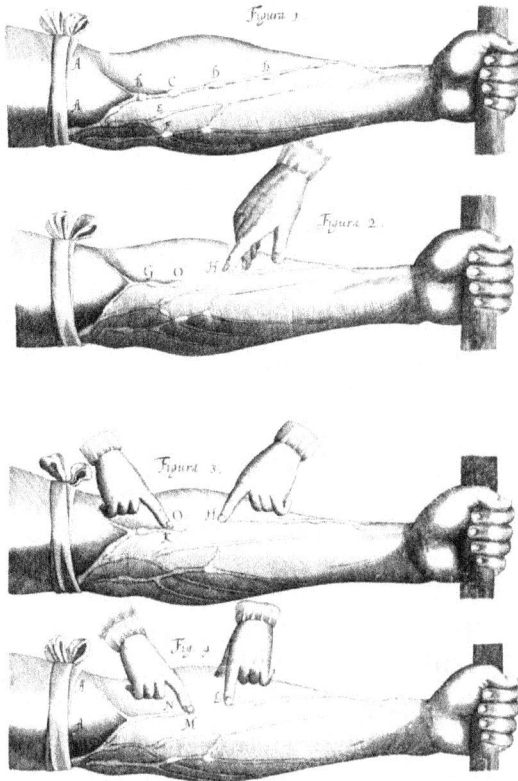

A mixed reaction greeted Harvey's masterpiece. Galenists did not hesitate to condemn his approach, even though his book is saturated with the ideas of Galen and Aristotle. Some even went so far as to claim that if dissection had proven Galen wrong, then nature had meanwhile changed! Guy Patin, dean of the Paris Faculty of Medicine called Harvey's theory *"paradoxical, useless, false, impossible, absurd and harmful."* Other voices came to his defense, however. René Descartes (1596-1650), the great French philosopher, immediately supported Harvey, stating unequivocally that blood in the body was in a state of perpetual circulation.[4]

_____

[4] Descartes, too, derived his practical knowledge mostly from the dissection of animal specimens. His posthumous book *De homine* (1662) was one of the first textbooks on physiology. There one also finds a mechanistic description of the pneuma - *The cavities of the brain are central reservoirs ... animal spirits enter these cavities. They pass into the pores of its substance and from these pores into the nerves. The nerves may be compared to the tubes of a waterworks; breathing or other actions depend on the flow of animal spirits into the nerves. The rational soul (the pineal) takes place of the engineer, living in that part of the reservoir that connects*

Descartes' opinion must be seen in light of his highly mechanistic approach to the subject of human physiology. He read into Harvey's discoveries further confirmation of his mechanistic views. Harvey, on the other hand, a convinced Aristotelian, opposed this view, adhering instead to a traditional, vitalistic view that held that life had special qualities over and above those of simple matter. Following Aristotle, he believed the heart to be the central organ of the body and the blood to be the principle of life. For Harvey, the beat of the heart was a manifestation of the soul vested in it, while Descartes held the view that the heart acted mechanically.

Paracelsians and the Iatrochemical School of Medicine

We are not only born and nourished by the means of Ferments; but we also Dye; Every Disease acts its Tragedies by the strength of some Ferment. For either the Sulphureous and Spirituous part of the blood, being too much carried forth, boyls up immoderately in the Vessels, like Wine growing hot, and from thence Feavers of a divers kind and nature are enkindled: or sometimes the Saline part of the blood, being carried forth, suffers a flux; and from thence it being made acid, austere and sometimes sharp, is apt for various Coagulations; from which the Scurvy, Dropsie, Stone, Leprosie, and many Chronical Diseases arise. (Willis)

The theories of Paracelsus promoted increased interest in the study of the chemical basis of all natural phenomena, not only those related to human health and disease. The existence of a central fire deep in the earth; the growth of metals; the origin of volcanoes, hot water springs, and mountain streams; the gaseous makeup of the atmosphere; and even questions concerning agriculture - were subjects intensely studied by 'iatrochemists' and others. This more general effort helped stimulate the development of new chemical methods that were used in the search for new drugs.

By the 1550s Paracelsus' writings and ideas were making their way across Europe and gaining increasing attention, not least of which was caused by the violence with which his enemies attacked his works. Controversy surrounded both his occult interpretations of the universe as well as his emphasis on new chemicals for treating disease. For the traditional Galenists, Paracelsus was a dangerous innovator who advocated lethal poisons for medicines. The use of

---

all of the various tubes. These spirits are like the wind. When they flow into a muscle they cause it to become stiff and harden, just as air in a balloon makes it hard.

36

antimony, for example, which Paracelsus used under the name of stibium as an emetic and purgative in the treatment of certain fevers, became a cause célèbre in France in the early 17th century, seriously dividing the medical community.

Nothing could stop the circulation of the reports of his remarkable cures for a variety of diseases, including syphilis and gout. And as these reports circulated greater attention was given to the use of chemical remedies; many became incorporated in medical textbooks published at the end of the 16th and beginning of the 17th centuries. All of this corresponded in time to when chemistry (as opposed to alchemy) was beginning to emerge as an independent and reputable field of study.

Johann Baptista van Helmont (1579-1644) was an important Paracelsian. The 1876 Encyclopedia Britannica qualified him as *"an excentric genius, (who) constructed a medical system which had some practical merits, (applied) therapeutical methods (that) were mild and in many respects happy, and (applied) newer chemical methods to the preparation of drugs."* His *"mild medicine was a reaction against the enormous and often lethal dosing of his time."* He was perhaps the last to claim to have made gold from lead!

Van Helmont was born in Brussels, came of a noble family and was educated at Louvain. He attended courses in magic and mystical philosophy organized by the Jesuits, toyed with the idea of joining the Capuchin order, and gave courses in surgery in the Medical College at Louvain at the age of seventeen. He became a physician in 1599. However, he lost his faith in medicine as then practiced following the treatment and advice received from two physicians when he fell seriously ill while on a long voyage. He decided to *"renounce the errors of the schools concerning what they rashly regarded as the groundwork of medicine."* From 1609 on he dedicated himself to the Paracelsian goal of using alchemy to discover new treatments and in the process to demolish the whole ancient system of elements, humors and their qualities.

Although strongly influenced by the works and mystical philosophy of Paracelsus, van Helmont charted his own course of study. He rejected both the four elements of Aristotle as well as the three substances of Paracelsus. Instead, he came to see *water* as the **only** material substance. As an inert and 'empty' medium, water became something else by the addition of 'spiritual' matter.

His own experiments confirmed the importance of water. He placed two hundred pounds of carefully dried earth in an earthen pot, in which he planted a five-pound willow tree. He covered the pot to prevent any material escaping or being added to the pot. He only supplied the pot with water over a period of five years, at the end of which the tree weighed one hundred sixty-nine pounds and three ounces, while the earth, after drying, was found to have lost two ounces. Water alone, it would seem, accounted for the gain of one hundred and sixty-four pounds. He had developed his own balance to achieve such precise weighing.

When van Helmont heated sixty-two pounds of coal in a closed vessel he found one pound deposited as ash and the rest had formed a smoke that was neither water nor air. He named this substance *gas* (derived from the Greek *chaos*, as used by Paracelsus in the general sense of air). In later experiments he was to find fifteen different gases including what would later be shown to be carbon dioxide, a gas that he called *gas sylvestre*.

For van Helmont, gasses represented a spiritual quality of matter that he called the *archeus*. God had endowed all matter - animals, vegetables and minerals - with this soul-like spirit. There were spirits celestial, infernal, human, metal, mineral and salt, spirits in herbs, roots and wood, flesh, blood, bones, and so on.

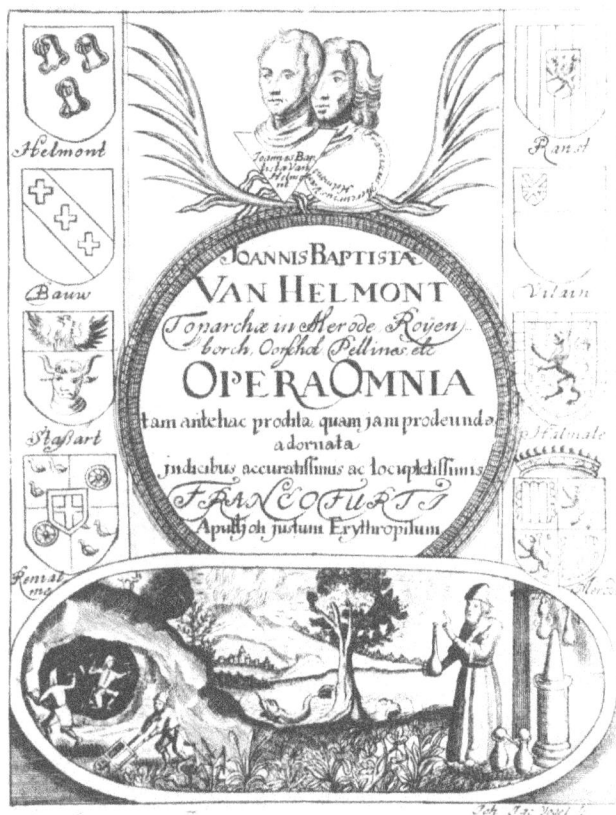

Closely linked with gas were ferments. Fermentation was known to the ancients and was strongly associated with yeast-like effervescence and bubbling. Alchemists invoked ferments when interaction between two or more components produced something new. Van Helmont's ferments were endowed with spiritual properties in keeping with their individual archei. He contributed significantly to the elucidation of the role of an acid ferment in gastric digestion. His experiments led him to believe that the pyloric opening of the stomach was the most sensitive bodily archeus. On one occasion, after having swallowed aconite (monkshood), he *"felt himself thinking in his stomach."*

Having endowed all objects and bodies with their own unique archeus, van Helmont's interpretation of disease and treatment differed radically from the ancients and even somewhat from Paracelsus. He replaced the ancient notion of humoral imbalance with archei that disturbed normal functioning of the body, or as he put it - *"a strange guest received within and endowed with a more powerful or able archeus.*" He allowed for the possibility that there were distinct diseases that could be distinguished by the different manner in which they penetrated and irritated the affected archeus. But where Paracelsus imagined that undigested and dead tartar deposits caused morbid responses, van Helmont claimed that the response was the consequence of a dynamic engagement between the archeus of the foreign guest and that of the host. He even saw fever in terms of the hosts defense reaction and not in morbific terms as the Galenists had.

It followed from his logic that treatment had to help that part of the body that was affected fight off the invading 'guest'. There was much less room in this logic for bloodletting or purges. Instead, herbs and minerals were his preferred means for treating illnesses.

Franciscus Sylvius (1614-1672), who was born in Hanau, Germany, is considered the real founder of the doctrine of 'iatrochemistry', which represented a kind of compromise between humoral pathology and the ideas of Paracelsus and van Helmont. Many of his chemical theories represented those of van Helmont stripped of their spiritual underpinnings. According to his theory, an individual's health depended on the maintenance of both a quantitative and qualitative balance of the alkaline and acid substances in the body. These substances were produced by a variety of transformations in the body, which involved what he too called ferments. Fermentation was supposed to take place in the stomach and played an important part in the body's vital processes. An acrimony or excess of either the acid or the alkaline substances, or their being in the wrong place, caused fevers and other diseases. They needed to be treated by drugs that had a contrasting nature, i.e. acidic drugs for excess alkaline and alkaline drugs for excess acid. The remedies he employed were partly Galenical, partly chemical.[5]

---

[5] Legend has it that Sylvius blamed God for the death of many of his patients that he had treated during an epidemic with 'appropriate' remedies. God, he said, had chosen to punish them for their sins by withholding His blessing.

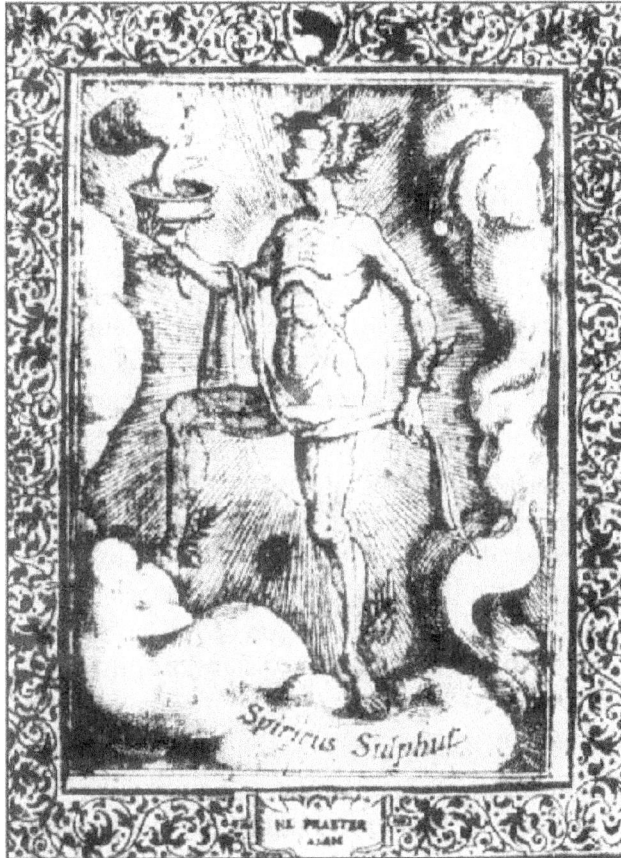

Spiritus Sulphur

The English physician Thomas Willis (1621-1675), who in fact had interpreted fever as fermentation before Sylvius, accepted Sylvius' chemical conception of disease. Although Willis started out believing only in Galen's humoral theories, he ended up favoring the Paracelsian doctrine that regarded all bodies, organic and inorganic, as composed of the elements - spirit, sulfur, salt, water and earth. He saw all fermenting bodies as being composed of these elements; it is the struggling and straining of each against the others that cause the movement in fermentation. When this occurs in the blood, it gives rise to a fever, as described in the opening quote above.

In the preface to his book on fevers *De febribus* published in 1660, Willis indicates that it was Harvey's discovery of circulation that led him to discard humoralist doctrine. No longer could the blood be seen as stagnating in the vessels. This long-accepted Galenic belief had played a critical role in the description of many diseases, particularly those involving fevers. Willis elaborated a rational approach to the use of drugs based on this new chemical view of the body. This appeared in his *Pharmaceutice Rationalis*, which had great influence in its time.[6] Willis was a member of the small group of learned men who gave birth to the Royal Society in 1660.

While the three principles of Paracelsus gained ground among the iatrochemists and pharmacists during the course of the 17th century, most believers, including Willis, were forced to add one or two other elements to account for new observations. For example, where distillations gave rise to heavier liquids and insoluble solids, the 'passive' elements of phlegm and earth were added. This gave rise to the concept of five elements, although there was never any real agreement among investigators as to the precise nature of the two elements required to make a complete set.

A variant view of certain diseases arose from a line of study that built on Paracelsus' interests in the medicinal benefits of thermal baths. Seeing the earth as a vast chemical laboratory, later Paracelsians suggested that the Earth's heat, as manifested in thermal baths, volcanoes and the underground formation of metals, resulted from a reaction of sulfur and a nitrous salt in the earth. This suggested to the French Paracelsian Joseph Duchesne (1544-1609) that diseases characterized by hot and burning qualities resulted from the inhalation of aerial sulfur and niter.

One critical outcome from all of these investigations was the inadequacy of the Aristotelian theory of forms and matter that had so dominated thinking up until then. Aristotle's theories required that all changes involved a transmutation, i.e. some fundamental change in one of the 'virtues' or hidden 'qualities' of a substance, e.g. the 'form' of whiteness that gave rise to the color of white. It was these qualities, in fact, that later became known as 'occult', because they could not be sensed directly. Aristotle's theories virtually made it impossible to recover the same matter after it had undergone a chemical change, and yet that is precisely what one experiment after another obtained in the mid 17th century.

The complexity of the changes observed so stressed the five-element concept, that it was forced to yield to newer notions, ones that conceived of matter in

---

[6] The great Canadian physician, Sir William Osler (1849-1919) was later to say about this work: "*It is as dead as Willis. It gives me a shudder to think of the constitution our ancestors had, and of how they withstood the assaults of the apothecary.*"

atomistic terms, some-what along the lines of the Greek atomists, that Galen had severely castigated.

Boyle's Corpuscles and the Iatrophysical School of Medicine

I have endeavored to deliver matters of fact so faithfully, that I may as well assist the lesse skillful readers to examine the chymical hypothesis, as provoke the spagirical (alchemical) philosophers to illustrate it...(Boyle)

The particulate, atomistic view of nature grew in parallel with the chemical developments just described. This view did not attempt any new explanation of chemical properties. Instead, it attempted to explain physiological and pathological processes in mechanical terms. For example, Pierre Gassendi (1592-1655), a close friend of Descartes, imagined that heat was due to small, round atoms, and cold, to pyramidal atoms with sharp points, which accounted for the pricking sensation of severe cold. Solids were held together by interlocking hooks. Descartes, on the other hand, preferred the motion of atoms to their shape.

Robert Boyle (1627-1691) played an important role in resurrecting the place of atomic/corpuscular theory of matter in medicine. Even though he himself was not a physician, he paid great attention to the medical usefulness of his ideas and discoveries, advocating what some would call today a multidisciplinary holistic approach to the practice of medicine, one involving not only trained physicians but chemists and other natural philosophers as well.

Boyle learned to speak Latin and French early in childhood and was only eight when he was sent to Eton where it is said he gained a passion for learning. He was brought up in a strong Calvinist environment and remained deeply religious throughout his life. He believed on several occasions that he felt directly the workings of a divine guidance. At age thirteen, on one such occasion he decided that *"his life should be more religiously and watchfully employed."* Upon his return to England in 1644, following six years on the Continent, he began a serious study of the Christian religion, became involved with a group of scholars studying natural philosophy, and started reading the works of Copernicus and Gassendi, among others. It was these readings, particularly Gassendi's efforts to present atomistic ideas in a form palatable to Christian theology, that led him to become interested in exploiting chemistry for its practical usefulness and because it could *"lead to a deeper understanding of God and Nature."* Boyle, following in the footsteps of Francis Bacon (1561-1626), attempted to keep separate his religious beliefs from his natural philosophy. He explained empirical results in a scientific manner; in doing so, he conceived the workings of the human body without resorting to spiritual intermediaries.

Later in life, Boyle became a close friend of Thomas Sydenham (1624-1689), a practicing physician in London. Sydenham allowed Boyle to accompany him in attending patients and there are many indications that when asked Boyle did not hesitate to offer medical advice. He received an honorary degree of 'doctor of physick' from Oxford in 1665.

Boyle was aware of the works of Paracelsus and van Helmont, since it was around 1650 that works of both had been translated into English by those interested in the application of chemistry in medicine. Also, the works of Paracelsus and other German mystics were being used to support the Puritan cause in England and related calls for reform of the medical establishment. Traditional Galenic training was judged on one hand too 'pagan' and on the other hand too 'popist'. Paracelsian medicine was the obvious remedy.

Boyle was deeply impressed by the experimental works of the *"bold and ingenious"* van Helmont. He confirmed van Helmont's willow-tree experiment using the more rapidly growing squash plant and accepted that *"all Vegetables do materially arise wholly out of the Element of water."* For a while he toyed with the idea that water was the ultimate principle in nature but ended up rejecting it because *"Helmont gives us no instance of the production of minerals out of water"* but instead relies on the *"operations of the alkahest...,"* a term invented by Paracelsus to denote a universal solvent. Significantly, Boyle justified his rejection by noting that the *"operations of the alkahest ... cannot be satisfactorily examined by you and me."*[7]

As presented in great and convincing detail in his *The Sceptical Chymist*, Boyle's own laboratory experience convinced him that neither the ancient Greek four elements nor the more recent three principles of Paracelsus were founded on verifiable experiments. If they (current adherents to either of

---

[7] This did not keep Boyle himself from seeking to discover the alkahest. He, like Paracelsus and van Helmont, believed that his deep faith in God would be rewarded by greater accomplishments. While most of his alchemical papers were destroyed by his editors, evidence of his 'quest' has been documented. Boyle, himself, claimed that he had transmutated gold into silver.

these theories) had tried to confirm their theories, *"they would, as well as I, have found them not to be true."* Worse, they don't cite the name or names of those who have supposedly carried out each of the experiments reported on. If they were at least to do that, *"they would secure themselves from the suspicion of falsehood ... and they would leave the reader to judge of what is fit for him to believe of what is delivered."*

Although he was not yet fully ready to address the question of what matter is made of, he did propose the existence of *"little particles of several sizes and shapes variously moved ... (that) were here and there associated into minute masses and clusters, and did by their coalitions constitute great store of such little primary concretions and masses as were not easily dissipable into such particles as composed them."* These he saw as *"distinct substances"* which could *"without very much inconvenience be called elements or principles."*

In 1671 Boyle published his *Tracts about the Cosmical Qualities of Things* in which he laid out his basic principles of matter. Matter, he wrote, is divided into finite parts that are produced by local motion while being made up of smaller, insensible particles called *"corpuscles."* These corpuscles aggregated to make up a mass or body, but in doing so, generally left space between one composed mass and another. Therefore, almost all solid bodies *"and some fluid ones that are made up of grosser parts"* have pores. Through these pores, there could enter what Boyle labeled *"effluviums,"* i.e., particles that separate from the bodies to which they belong because of some agitation of one kind or another, e.g. the heating up of a body.

Boyle rejected Paracelsus' and van Helmont's spiritual archei and replaced them with *"local motion"*:

> *If we fancy any two of the bodies about us, as a stone, a metal, &c. to have nothing at all to do with any other body in the universe, it is not easy to conceive either how one can act on the other, but by local motion (of the whole body or its corporeal effluvia); or how by motion it can do any more than put the parts of the other body into motion too, and thereby produce in them a change of situation and texture, or of some other of its mechanical affectations ...*

Local motion ensured that matter could fulfill its purpose **without** constant recourse to an external spirit or force; the insensitivity of corpuscles derived from his assumption that the smallest particles behaved mechanically, and had no ability to interact chemically.[8] Most motion derived from those laws that God had established at the time of Creation; however, on rare occasions, it could result from direct divine intervention.

The particulate, mechanistic approach to nature contributed to the rise of what came to be known as the iatrophysical school of medicine. This school introduced different ideas concerning the origin of diseases. For example, Gian Alfonso Borelli (1608-1679) of Naples, who is considered one of the founders of this school, believed that defective movements of the particles that made up the body caused fevers, pains and convulsions. He argued that the retention and rotting of oily, salty and watery particles among muscle fibers gave rise to abscesses, gout and *"other bad effects."* Furious agitation of the circulatory system (as placed in evidence by Harvey) provoked not only the wide circulation of these particles but their escape from the arteries. Giorgio Baglivi (1668-1706), known as 'the Italian Hippocrates', considered the body to be made of 'fibers' whose tension or relaxation caused disease. Archibald Pitcairn (1652-1713) considered that fever was caused by an acceleration of the blood flow, and William Cole (1635-1716) imagined that intermittent fevers were due to the blockage of the nerve root pores of the cerebral cortex.

These and many other explanations were introduced into pathology to explain the processes of fever and disease. They sometimes led to dramatically different treatments, especially if and when to use bloodletting and purgatives. However, by and large, Galenic medicine still dominated practice at the end of the 17th century, with the incorporation of new therapeutic products that had been introduced by the iatrochemists.

Return to the Hippocratic Bedside

... for after I had not found in Books what might satisfie a mind desirous of Truth, I resolved with my self, to search into living and breathing Examples: and therefore sitting often times by the Sick, I was wont carefully to search out their Cases, to weigh all the Symptoms, and to put them, with exact Diaries of the Diseases, into Writing ... (Willis)

---

[8] Recognising that he might be seen as limiting what God could or could not do, he added that each such particle *"though it be mentally, and by divine Omnipotence divisible, yet by reason of its smallness and solidity, nature doth scarce ever actually divide it."*

Willis, although one of the leading advocates of a chemical interpretation of physiological and pathological processes, was forced, as suggested by the quote above published in 1660, to acknowledge that he did not know enough to treat his patients well. The total failure of any system of treatment to alter the course of the Great Plague of London in 1665 provided further proof of the inadequacy of existing schools of medicine. There followed a general call from all leading physicians to a return to the Hippocratic bedside. Sydenham is given greatest credit, historically, for this movement.

Known as the 'English Hippocrates', Sydenham followed his ancient master in advocating a careful and accurate description of illnesses. A friend of the philosopher-physician John Locke (1632-1704), he also receives the greatest credit for reviving the Hippocratic notion of the 'epidemic constitution of the atmosphere', as discussed in Chapter III.

Sydenham's writings are far better known than the events of his life. He along with his father and brothers were deeply involved in the Civil War and for a while Sydenham seemed to be tempted by a political career. He only decided to devote his energies seriously to medicine around 1660. He did not obtain his MD, however, until 1676. He placed observation above everything, which led Locke to say of him:

> *You cannot imagine how far a little observation carefully made by a man not tied up to the four humors (Galen), or sal, sulphur, and mercury (Paracelsus), or to acid and alcali (Sylvius and Willis) which has of late prevailed, will carry a man in the curing of diseases though very stubborn and dangerous; and that with very little and common things, and almost no medicine at all.*

Locke particularly celebrated Sydenham's qualities as a healer. Following Hippocrates, Sydenham believed in the self-healing tendencies of the body and practiced conservative (cooling) treatment, lots of fluids and moderate bleeding. He based this treatment mostly on experience, not theory. Although a Puritan, he did not hesitate to promote the use of cinchona bark - 'the Jesuit powder' - against prevailing fevers and other diseases. Strictly orthodox physicians, however, refused to prescribe a remedy unknown to Galen. That it cured without producing any of the 'evacuations' claimed necessary by

Galen only added further evidence of the incompatibility of modern and Galenic pharmacological and pathological theories.[9]

* * * * *

Although iatrochemical and iatrophysical disease theories would in time be almost totally discarded, each of the physicians cited above contributed to the real advancement of physiological knowledge. For example, van Helmont discovered the importance of the gastric sac in the digestive process.[10] Sylvius was the first to describe the tubercles in patients suffering from phthisis (tuberculosis). He and his followers added considerably to the knowledge of physiological processes, notably by examining the digestive fluids, such as saliva, gastric juices and the secretions of the pancreas. Borelli contributed to an understanding of the function of the intercostal muscles and the diaphragm in breathing. Willis was the first to note the sweetish taste of diabetic urine. He gave excellent descriptions of puerperal fever, typhoid fever (see Chapter IV), and hysteria. He was one of the first to regard hysteria as a disease of the nervous system. Sydenham left classic descriptions of gout, influenza, measles, rheumatic fever, and scarlet fever (see Chapter IV).

One of the interesting features of the physical theories developed in the 17th century is their resemblance to the some of the theories of ancient Greece - the particles of Boyle smack of the atoms of Democritus and molecules of Asclepiades - the need to relax the bodies' fibers and keep the body fluids in motion would have fitted perfectly in the approaches advocated by the Methodist school.

---

[9] The new iatrochemical theories, as expressed by Willis, explained the action of the cinchona bark in terms of how bark particles mix with the blood and force it into a new fermentation, whose continual agitation prevents the blood from accumulating dregs or feverish swellings.

[10] Van Helmont's discovery of gastric acid digestion demonstrated that organic growth is a process of 'addition'. This undermined the Galenic concept of heat and cooking (coction) and played an important part in disproving Aristotelian notions concerning organic growth.

ARGVMENTVM MARSILII FI-
CINI FLORENTINI IN LIBRū
MERCVR II TRISMEGISTI AD
COSMVM MEDICEM PATRIAE
PATREM.

O tēpore:quo Moyſes natus
eſt:floruit Athlas aſtrologus
Promethei phiſici frater. ac
maternus auus maioris Mer-
curii : cuius nepos fuit Mercurius Triſme-
giſtus. Hoc autem de illo ſcribit Aurelius
Auguſtinus.Quāq̃ Cicero:aeq̃ Lactantius:
Mercurios quinq̃ per ordinē fuiſſe uolūt.
quintumq̃ fuiſſe illum:qui ab ægyptiis
        :a grecis autē Triſmegiſtus appel-
latus eſt.Hunc aſſerunt occidiſſe argū:ægi
ptiis præfuiſſe:eiſq̃ leges:ac lƒas tradidiſſe.
Litterarum uero caracteres in animaliū ar-
borumq̃ figuris inſtituiſſe.Hic in tanta ho-
minum ueneratiōe fuit:ut in deoꝝ numerū
relatus ſit.Templa illius numinis cōſtructa
q̃plurima.Nomen eius proprium:ob reuerē
tiam quandam pronūtiare:uulgo ac temere

III

On the Origin of Epidemics

From the 14th century onwards, with plague being the outstanding example of the time, Europe was confronted with one epidemic after another. The populace at large had its own interpretations as to the causes of these catastrophes, but physicians were the ones that were expected to provide authoritative opinions based on their deeper knowledge of natural philosophy. We have already seen at the end of Chapter I and in Chapter II that in some medical circles the conceptualization of disease had undergone a radical change from the time of Hippocrates and Galen. In this Chapter we examine these changes a bit more closely with the aim of obtaining a clearer picture on how epidemics were viewed by physicians prior to the 18th century.

Neo-Platonic, Religious and Other 'Occult' Influences

Magic has power to experience and fathom things which are inaccessible to human reason. For magic is a great secret wisdom ...

All skills and arts are from God, and nothing comes from any other source ... and therefore no one may vilify astronomy, alchemy, or medicine, or philosophy, or theology, acting poetry, music geomancy ... or any other high art. (Paracelsus)

Astronomy, by which Paracelsus meant astrology, along with alchemy have long histories in the practice of the healing arts. Astrology probably began as a phase of animism whereby the sun, moon, stars and planets were regarded as living beings. It was the ancient Greeks who extended the scope of astrology, connecting it with practically all of the known sciences, including medicine. As the motions of astral bodies were more accurately charted, and heaven and earth were inextricably connected along the lines suggested by Plato and the Neo-Platonists, there grew the belief that these bodies controlled the fate of the entire universe.

The Hippocratic Corpus, as already noted, did not pay any great heed to astrology, nor did Galen, although he did ascribe some importance to the position of the planets in the determination of when to treat and when to expect crises to occur. More important was the preservation by Arabic scholars of the astronomical discoveries of their predecessors and the extension of observations and mathematical methods, including the introduction, from India, of our present system of writing numbers.

The medical writings of the major Arabic physicians were translated into Latin beginning in the 13th century and were used in medical schools for several centuries. Rhazes (865-925), for example, said of astrology:

> *Wise men among the* medici *agree that everything relating to times, the air, and waters, and complexions, and diseases is changed by the motion of the planets.*

Thus it is not surprising that when medieval theorists had to explain why plague had assumed such appalling proportions in 1348 they relied on a celestial explanation. The Paris Faculty determined that on March 20, 1345, at one-o'clock PM, there had occurred a conjunction of Mars, Jupiter and Saturn in the sign of Aquarius. That, with other conjunctions and eclipses, was the whole cause of the trouble. Jupiter had drawn up evil vapors from the earth and water; and Mars, a malevolent planet that generated choler and wars, was from October 6, 1347, to May 1348 in the constellation of the Lion together with the head of the Dragon. Mars, being on the wane, was particularly active in drawing up vapors and, since its evil aspect was turned towards Jupiter, a disposition or quality hostile to human life was engendered. No magic was part of this explanation, only naturalist phenomena!

Going on in this vein, the reason why the epidemic raged in two distant towns and not in places between them was "*on account of the aspects and rays of the planets which strike these places, like the glance of the eyes upon an object; as Saturn looks upon Mars with malignant aspect, or Mars with malignant aspect upon humane Jupiter, then the rays of those planets kill where they strike.*"

Similarly, Ficino, in his plague manuscript *Consiglio contro la pestilentia* published in 1481, indicated that the "*poisonous vapor*" that had given rise to plague had formed "*under maligned constellations, mostly at a conjunction of Mars with Saturn.*" This vapor "*resembles a vital spirit*" and is harmful "*because its mixture is directly contrary in proportion to the composition of the vital spirit of the heart.*" However, such a vapor can only arise when the air has been contaminated by miasmatic influences. Furthermore, it cannot penetrate the human body "*if the humors are not open to fever.*" Therefore, wrote Ficino, "*you must correct the air, purge the humors, and fortify the heart.*"

It was well known that decaying matter could contaminate the air. The Paris Faculty concluded that decaying matter piled up in the interior of the earth until it caused an earthquake, which released this corrupted matter into the air. Of more immediate importance were emanations from lakes and ponds, evil-smelling putrefactions of dead bodies of men or animals, and putrid fumes from manure and rotting plants and vegetables, all of which Hippocrates had identified earlier.

Ficino was probably not your typical physician of the late 15th century, in that he was more a philosopher and man of letters than a practicing doctor. Nevertheless, health and the practical side of medicine occupied an important place in his writings. Furthermore, his father was a respected and popular Florentine surgeon/doctor and his own medical education was obtained from the University of Bologna, one of the oldest (founded in 1158) and most reputable medical schools in Europe. Italian medical schools were generally notable for their strong medical-astrological culture. Many practicing physicians often combined their medical and astrological practice, especially in the service of princes.

Ficino spent much of his life translating and interpreting Plato and Neo-Platonists, as well as formulating and diffusing his own Christianized version of Platonic philosophy. He was encouraged to pursue this direction by the Greek cardinal Basil Bessarion's (1403-72) acceptance of Plato as a 'precursor of Christ'. Ficino also introduced into Christian thinking the manuscript *Corpus Hermeticum*, a work supposedly written by Hermes Trismegistus, who purportedly lived around the time of Moses. This text was one of many Hellenic manuscripts brought to Italy by Byzantine scholars who had fled Constantinople after it fell to the Turks in 1453.

The Egyptian religious beliefs spelled out in the *Corpus* seemed to be precursors to what Plato would later say, and they prophesized the coming of Christ, 'the Son of God'. As a result the whole work was treated with great reverence and intensely studied into the 17th century even well after it was shown in 1614 to be a compilation of different writers who had lived during the first few centuries **after** Christ.

Ficino believed Hermes to be "*the first philosopher to raise himself above physics and mathematics to the contemplation of the divine ...*" He incorporated much of Hermes' thinking in his best-selling *Book of Life* written in 1489. With Hermes on his side, Ficino dared to add magic to his medicine bag, although phrased in such a way as to avoid, just barely, any accusation of heresy. Augustine, who knew of the Hermetic writings and equally believed them to have been written "*long before the sages and philosophers of Greece,*" attacked the work for praising the magic used by the Egyptians to draw spirits and demons into the statues of their gods, thereby purportedly animating them. Ficino, as editor to the translations, was successful in using Augustine's name to certify the acceptability of this work, while not making known Augustine's criticism!

The writings of Hermes played a major role in reviving and legitimizing the use of and belief in occult forces for medical purposes. The cosmos was conceived in terms of a tightly knit relationship between heaven and earth, one which could be controlled by those who knew how to canalize the effluvia and influences pouring down onto the earth from the stars. It was sometimes necessary to call upon *decans*, which were seen as possessing powerful divine or demonic forces. These forces were best channeled by the use of talismans, images of stars inscribed on the correct materials, at the right times and in the right frame of mind.

Ficino proposed the use of amulets, talismans and charms, on which astral images would be carved showing a suitable heavenly spirit to acquire "*medicines from the heavens.*" For those who wear them, these images "*have a power against harmful things, like poisons or plague.*" Ficino took great care to note that he was thinking of planetary talismans to be used following "*spiritual*" magic and not in the "*demonic*" manner. The image could be made in brass, combined with gold and silver, the metals of Jupiter, Sol, and Venus.

Although the use of amulets may be the oldest form of prophylaxis against disease, Hippocrates had found no place in his medicine for them or any other form of magic such as charms or incantations. But, as already noted, his efforts to dissociate medicine from spiritual influences had totally failed. Ficino provides us with yet another example of such failure when he wrote "*on the power of words and songs in obtaining heavenly gifts and on the seven steps leading to the celestial things.*" Here we find Ficino at his Hermetic best:

> *Harder materials, stones and metals, hold the lowest step, and these seem to refer to the Moon. The second place, in ascending order, belongs to things which are made from herbs, the fruits of trees, gums, and the limbs of animals, and these answer to Mercury, if we follow the heavenly order of the Chaldeans. In third place are the subtlest powders and the vapors selected from them, and the odors of herbs, flowers, and unguents pertaining to Venus. In fourth place are words, songs, and sounds, all of which are rightly dedicated to Apollo, the author of Music beyond all other*

things. In fifth place are the powerful concepts of the imagination, forms, movements, and affects, all having a Martial force. In sixth place are the discourses and deliberations of human reason, which belong to Jove. Seventh place is for more secret and simpler intelligences, almost separated now from movement, joined to divine things, and devoted to Saturn.

In applying these steps, the physician is to be guided by the parallel to be found between heavenly and bodily forms. Here Ficino is following in the footsteps of Plato and the Neo-Platonists that he had translated. It is the universal soul, the *anima mundi*, which served to link the macrocosm with the microcosm. Its power *"spreads out through all things"* and can be infused *"into those which draw its spirit the most."* By learning which part of the heavens corresponds to our bodily needs, we *"are able to lay claim to the heavenly bodies."*

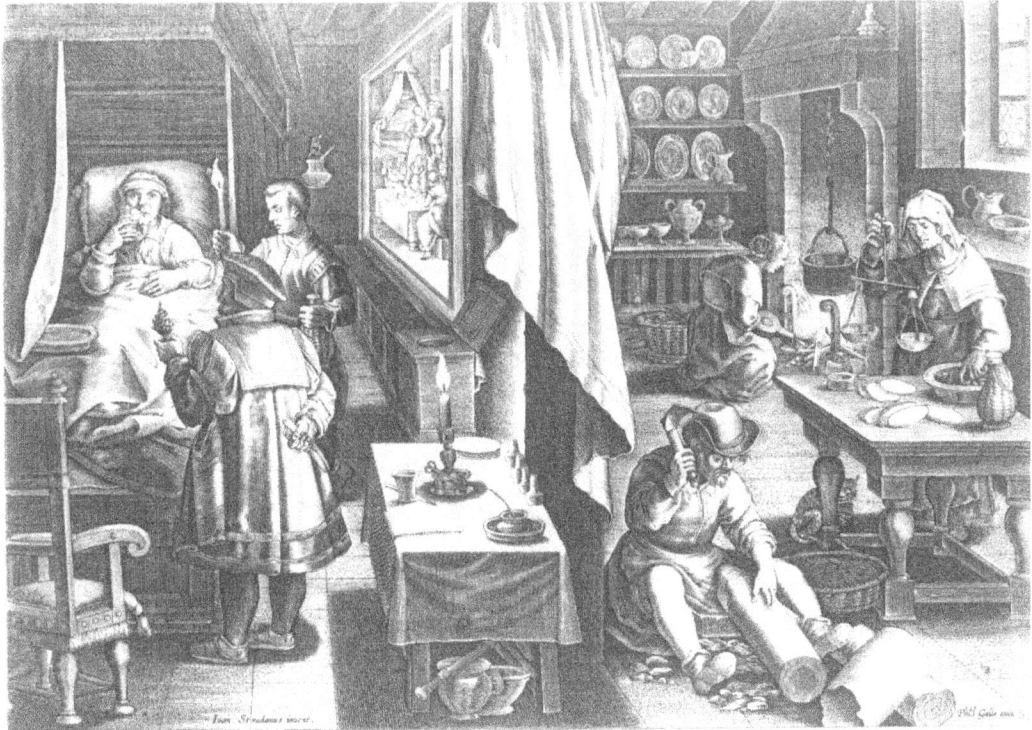

HYACVM, ET LVES VENEREA.

Grauata morbo ab hocce membra mollia   Leuabit ista forpta coctio arboris.

55

Thus:

> *If you want your body and spirit to receive power from some limb of the world, for example from the Sun, learn which are the Solar things among metals and stones, even more among plants ...*

Like Ficino, Paracelsus believed *"everything external in nature points to something internal; for nature is both inside man and outside man."* Since **all** matter had been shaped by the stars, it suggested the presence of powerful remedies in nature that corresponded to human diseases whose origins were also to be found in the stars, since *"there is nothing that nature has not signed in such a way that man may discover its essence."*

Paracelsus' approach to syphilis illustrates how he applied the principle of 'signatures'. The Galenists argued that the West Indian origin of guaiac justified its use for treating syphilis, a disease that also came from that part of the world. Syphilitic patients were placed in closed chambers where they were exposed to the vapors of burning guaiac. Paracelsus, however, reasoned that since syphilis was acquired from venal girls, it is 'signed' by the god of the market, Mercury, thus making it a 'mercurial' disease! So he came out on the side of 'metalism', i.e. the use of mercury, opposing the use of wood or any other product derived from the vegetable family.[11]

Paracelsus' belief in 'signatures' paralleled his adherence to the 'like-to-like' principle, another point that placed him at odds with the Galenists. Galen had called for driving out hot with cold, or moist with dry, while Paracelsus envisaged that the cure of disease was to be found in that which caused the disease. For example - *"whatever causes jaundice, also cures jaundice,"* and *"the physic which should cure paralysis must come from the same thing that caused the disease."* Like-to-like explained why a tartrate chemical could cure a disease like arthritis involving the accumulation of tartar.[12]

In applying both the signature and the like-to-like principles, Paracelsus rejected the humoral basis for disease, preferring instead external factors that introduce themselves into the body through the air, food or drink.

---

[11] Unfortunately for Paracelsus, economic interests also favored the use of guaiac and opposed that of mercury. This resulted in his not being able to publish a more extensive treatise concerning syphilis. Like most of his other writings, it was only published after his death.

[12] Maintaining that this substance is an acid deposit that *"burns like hell, and Tartarus is hell,"* he called it tartar.

Specifically, the Hermetic doctrine of the macrocosm and the microcosm suggested that different external astral 'seeds' corresponded to different organs. Furthermore, understanding disease in (al)chemical terms suggested to Paracelsus that each organ of the body had its own digestive process and that disease resulted from the inability of that process to digest whatever 'food' had been introduced externally to the body. Complicating matters was each person's specificity, a uniqueness guaranteed by the *"various moments at which we are born."* For *"if the same heaven were in all of us, all men would have to be equally sick and equally healthy."*

Moving into the 17th century, we find related beliefs still strongly entrenched in the extraordinary system of beliefs of Robert Fludd (1574-1637). Fludd was the son of Sir Thomas Fludd, Paymaster to the Forces in France and the Netherlands during the reign of Queen Elizabeth. His travels on the continent led him to learn about Paracelsus. There too he came across Ficino's translations of the work of Hermes Trismegistus. He obtained his degrees in medicine in 1605 but was several times rejected by the College of Physicians owing to his allegiance to Paracelsus. It was only in 1609 that his candidacy was finally accepted. He practiced medicine successfully in London until his death in 1637.

Fludd's major works, including the *History of the Macrocosm and the Microcosm* published in 1618, owed a considerable debt to Hermes.[13] In his books Fludd explained the creation of the universe in terms of God's active light filling the void wherever it fell. Where this light was strongest, less matter could exist. Only far away from heaven where the light was weakest, did the elemental world arise, made up of the traditional four states of matter - fire, air, water and earth. In between there was the ethereal world of stars and planets. The sun, placed as it were, at the midpoint in Fludd's 'Chain of Being' was very special since it was here where God had placed his tabernacle.[14]

---

[13] It was during Fludd's lifetime (1614) that Meric Casaubon demonstrated, through analysis of the text, that the *Hermetic Corpus* could not have been written by one person, and more importantly, that it had been written in the 2nd and 3rd centuries after the birth of Christ, facts that Fludd and many other Hermeticists were ignorant of or chose to ignore.

[14] Fludd wrote many hundreds of pages over a twenty year period in which these and related ideas were described. My description of his ideas is at best rather 'suggestive', an adjective that applies as well to the brief descriptions given of the ideas of Paracelsus and van Helmont.

Plague Legends

The universe was still actively under the influence of God. God, as chief chemist, carried out his transformations through the countless numbers of beings that inhabit his three worlds - the heavens with its hierarchy of angelic creatures, the ethereal with good and evil demons, and the elemental with men, animals, plants and minerals - "*God is in everything that existeth, seeing that from Him, by Him, and in Him are all things.*" Whereas most other Hermeticists seemed content to remain rather vague in describing the working of the universe, Fludd did not hesitate, both verbally and graphically, to give shape to the manner in which spiritual as well as demonic forces worked. In doing so, he drew upon many of the mechanistic interpretations that were then coming into vogue. Given that his writings span a period during which similar mechanistic principles were being developed and demonstrated, one could view Fludd's attempts at applying state-of-the-art thinking to a Hermetic universe.

Fludd firmly believed in a stationary Earth with planets rotating in a circular motion. This belief had supposedly led him to the idea that blood might circulate several years before his close friend Harvey was to come to that same conclusion. He was one of the first to publish support for Harvey's findings. Harvey, echoing Fludd's beliefs, conceived the relationship between the human heart and the sun as follows:

> The heart, consequently, is the beginning of life; the sun of the microcosm, even as the sun in his turn might well be designated the heart of the world.

In Fludd's world, all occult action, including sympathy and antipathy, is due to "*angelicall irridations or shinings.*" These extraterrestrial 'beams' touch all matter and things, which in turn emit their own beams, as illustrated by - "*Medicines do send forth their influences in beams.*" How individuals react to these beams is conditioned by the horoscope under which they were born.

Since the air "*itself is full of mystic and wonderful beings, souls, demons, angels, and other mysterious invisible existences,*" it follows that winds play a vital part in everyday life, including the health of individuals and whole communities. The winds are under the influence of four good angels and four bad angels. Each wind reveals a different characteristic of God; for example, one his clement side, another his severe side. What the winds impart is locally decided by the momentary action of demons and angels present. Fludd demonstrated this action by the phenomenon of expansion and contraction.

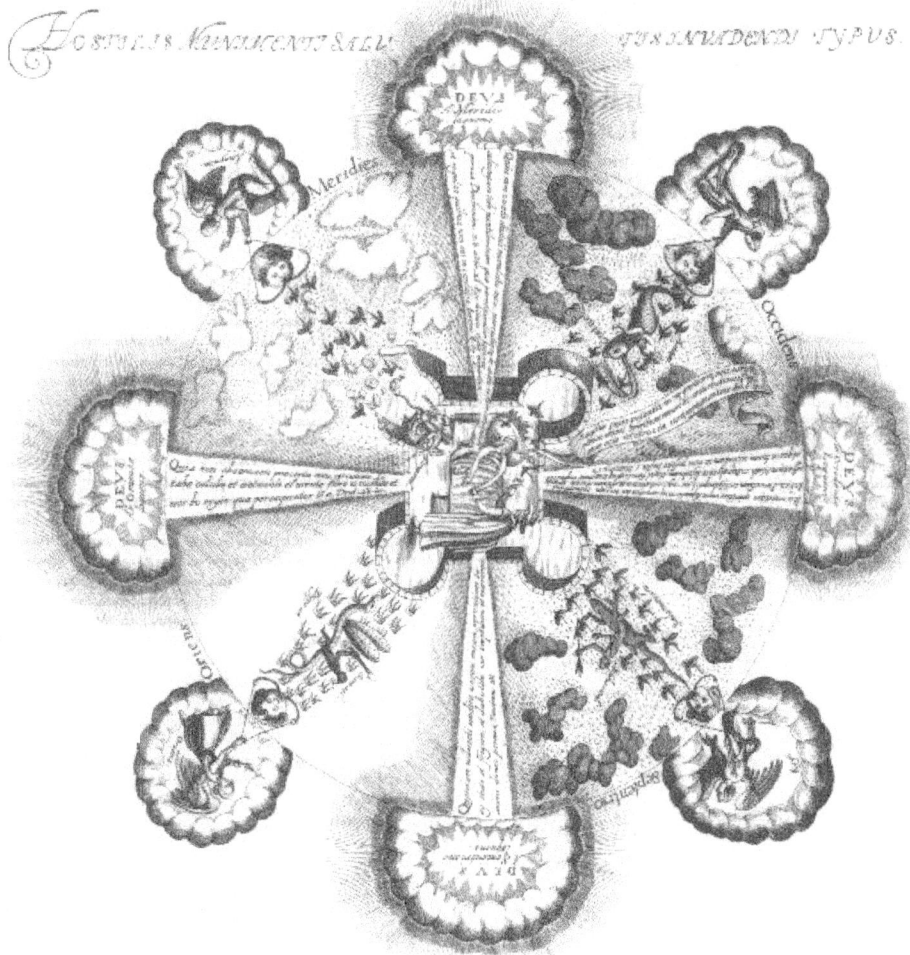

Using a form of thermometer-barometer, whose origin he claimed he found in the writings of Hermes, Fludd showed how the water level inside of an air-filled retort placed in a trough filled with water depended on the heat or coolness applied to the upper end of the retort. Since he, like Hermes, believed that everything consisted of one thing only - water, this devise illustrated how the demons and angels, acting on the outside of the body could affect the internal composition of the body. Demon-endowed moisture, for example, cause infections such as plague, measles, small pox and phthisis, while earthly substances in the atmosphere are associated with chronic infections as well as melancholy and stupor.

The winds were also responsible for certain physiological manifestations; thus, the east wind was the cause of an abnormal rise in temperature while the hard pulse was due to the north wind. Fludd, if nothing else, contributed to the notion that disease was a real thing, 'caused' by an external 'contagium' and not the result of internal abnormal mixture of the humors.

Fludd's eclectic system, which found room for the ancient humors, Hermetic astrology, Paracelsus' three substances and the recently discovered phenomenon of magnetism, did not seem to arouse any antagonism in England. Even Harvey, a staunch Aristotelian who irreverently called Paracelseans *"shit-breeches,"* was his friend. This largely reflected the degree of medical toleration that prevailed in England at the beginning of the 17th century, before the onset of civil unrest that culminated later in a civil war.

While Galenism and anti-Galenism began to take on a largely religious character in other parts of Europe, in England, a 'compromise' had been reached during the rule of Elizabeth I that, although essentially aimed to maintain peace among competing religious factions, allowed the so-called chemical doctors to practice and their new remedies to be accepted. The great majority of English physicians, however, paid no attention to the more occult aspects of Paracelsian thought and confined themselves to incorporating the new chemical remedies among their traditional Galenic ones.

While Fludd was tolerated in England, his work came under heavy attack on the Continent. Johannes Kepler (1571-1630), for example, engaged Fludd in an exchange of papers over a period of five years following the publication in 1618 of Fludd's *History* ....[15] Kepler practiced astrology and was very much a Neo-Platonist. They both sought 'harmony' in the universe. But Kepler worked with real measurements of planetary locations while Fludd had only words to play with. Kepler could not accept Fludd's use of geometry and mathematics to support pre-conceived macrocosm-microcosm analogies, and judged him to be *"enigmatic, emblematic and Hermetic."*

Equally opposed to Fludd's ideas were Marin Mersenne (1588-1648), Gassendi and interestingly enough van Helmont; interesting, because to the casual

---

[15]That Kepler took the time to correspond with Fludd is indicative of how well read Fludd was on the continent. It is especially remarkable given the fact that Kepler was forced to interrupt his studies in 1620 when his mother was arrested on a formal charge of witchcraft for which she was eventually acquitted but only after having spent 13 months in prison. She died in 1622 several months following her release.

observer both he and Fludd seemed to be promoting rather similar occult notions concerning physiology and the origin of diseases; but as we will explore shortly, this was not the case.

Mersenne was a priest who, operating out of his monastic cell in Paris, made it his business to know and correspond with the leading scientists of the time. He was in Paris in 1623 when the mysterious sect of the Rosicrucians visited to announce that they were in possession of many deep secrets concerning the art of treatment. Mersenne and his friends, that included Gassendi, were deeply concerned with the Hermetic influence on Christianity. They found this 'visitation' particularly alarming and initiated a propaganda war to attack the more prominent believers in Hermeticism. Top on the list of the accused was Fludd, who had earlier published several pieces in England defending Rosicrucian beliefs. In those works, Fludd had suggested that alchemy, natural magic and a 'new medicine' should replace Aristotle and Galen. Furthermore, since the vital spirit entered the body through inspiration, attention should be given to how this spirit nourished our bodies, in particular, how it entered and was dispersed through the arterial and venous systems.

Mersenne branded Fludd a heretic and a *"purveyor of stinking and horrible magic."* In his 1625 publication *La Vérité des Sciences* he devoted some four hundred pages to refute the claims of Fludd and other Hermeticists. Mersenne believed that the magic associated with Hermes was evil and would have fearful consequences if allowed to continue. In particular, it threatened his own mechanical and mathematical view of the universe, a view which his friend Descartes was soon to develop in a much more complete and authoritative fashion. If the views of Rosicrucians and Hermeticists were allowed to prevail, all phenomena would be explained by analogy between macrocosm and microcosm, stellar influences and the ever-present angels and demons.[16]

Mersenne did not oppose the experimental results of alchemy. In fact, he suggested the establishment of alchemical academies that would aim to improve the health of mankind. They would denounce charlatans, and

---

[16] Duchesne published a work in 1626 in which he showed by analogy how the vapors and exhalations rising from the lower regions of the brain become condensed in the same way that clouds and rains form from the earth and give rise to a cold and a runny nose. Winds, sleet, and snow might correspond to ringing in the ears, paralepsy and apoplexy.

discard allegorical and enigmatic terms replacing them with a clear terminology based upon laboratory operations. Van Helmont's work was judged to be sufficiently in the right direction to be acceptable. No doubt this contributed to the important place van Helmont had in the development of the iatrochemical school of medicine, as already described in Chapter II.

Van Helmont, who replied to Mersenne's campaign to vilify Fludd, accused Fludd of being a poor physician and a worse alchemist, and all-in-all a superficially learned man. He rejected the macro-microcosmic analogies so central to Fludd's (and Paracelsian) thinking. God did not act through the stars or any other intermediary, including amulets. Instead, God acted through the archei. This belief led van Helmont to religious confrontations that ended with his denunciation by the faculty at Louvain. Summoned by the Spanish Inquisition in 1623, much of his work was proclaimed heretical and he was confined to prison, and later, house arrest, only to be released in 1636. It would be another 6 years before formal proceedings against him were officially discontinued and he could return to publishing his ideas.

What got van Helmont into trouble was his 'magical' treatise on the *Magnetic Cure of Wounds*, published in 1621. This treatise reviewed the evidence concerning the pseudo-Paracelsian idea of a 'weapon-salve', a salve that was not applied directly to the wound but to the weapon that had inflicted it! Van Helmont criticized both those who had omitted the presence of thickened blood on the weapon and those who had argued that the salve had to have moss that came from the skull of a hanged criminal. Any skull would do including that from the head of a "*Jesuite, put to death by strangulation, or any other kinde of martyrdom.*" Van Helmont accused the Jesuits of being pseudo-scientific rhetoricians who interfered with the gathering of true knowledge by means of diligent study of nature.

William Gilbert (1544-1603), a firm believer in the theory that the world was alive, had published his epoch-making work on magnetism in 1600. For Kepler, magnetism accounted for celestial movements. For van Helmont, it provided an explanation for sympathetic healing, including the means whereby the salve on the weapon could act on a wound without having to touch it, or as he put it - "*the magnet is endowed with various senses and also with imagination, a certain Naturall phansy*". Its force was spiritual in nature and thus perfectly natural. His enemies, who had strong allies in Jesuit circles, argued that this magic was the work of the devil and thus heretical. Later Boyle rejected van Helmont's pamphlet on the magnetic cure of wounds. On the other hand, Boyle's corpuscular theory led him to accept the possibility that amulets might be beneficial.

During the long period that van Helmont was under home arrest, Fludd kept the weapon salve theory alive, incorporating it in his writings and defending it when attacked in 1632 by William Foster, an English country parson, for being *"magicall and unlawful."* Although Fludd was a close friend of Gilbert his explanation of how weapon salve worked followed traditional Hermetic theories. The blood in the wound and on the weapon *"doe sympathise together, even as wee see one thred extended from one end of a chamber unto the other."* Fludd claims to have successfully used this cure on several occasions. On one, he wiped the weapon clean on the second day of treatment and his patient suffered *"great paine"* that was relieved only when the salve was replaced. Fludd tore Foster's arguments to shreds. How, for example, could Foster believe that angels of heaven could not work their powers at a distance while those of hell could. And if Foster found it to be witchcraft, because it was not mentioned in the Holy Scripture, how could he not as well condemn *"causticke, viscicatory healing, fluxing, and other externall medicines daily used."*

Van Helmont replaced Fludd's Hermetic forces with ones that were equally challenging to the imagination. In Chapter II, the role of the archeus in gas and ferments was discussed. Not mentioned was the role of the archeus in the generation of ideas and images, and how such 'imagination' could affect other archei. For example, an image or idea could 'seed' a disease entity. While part of the explanation lies in the fear evoked by the threat of disease, especially when it is a disease as terrible as plague, van Helmont conceived a physical process to be involved as well. He made a particularly strong case for this form of causation in his analysis of allergies, especially asthma. He also ascribed the royal cure of scrofula as coming about through the power of the word to evoke the image and desire to be cured.

While van Helmont is still with us, we must note how his ideas supported belief in spontaneous generation. It helps to remember that he reduced all matter to only water; life, as such, is matter that is endowed with a working plan (spiritual directives) defining what it is to become. This plan can be altered by the action of odors and ferments. Spontaneous generation is just one possibility of an altered plan. This occurs in putrefied matter, as revealed by the odor connected with decay. Decay begins as a vague loosening of matter and is guided by the image of the object into which matter is to be transformed. This image together with odor constitutes the ferment, i.e. the vital principle of the new object.[17] Van Helmont's 'recipe' for the spontaneous generation of young mice was to place a jar of grain containing a dirty shirt in a warm place!

The belief in spontaneous generation was rather widespread among scientific circles of that time. Van Helmont invoked the involvement of a vital force. Boyle sidestepped the issue, calling instead upon 'exigencies' inherent in decaying matter. Spontaneous generation, wrote Boyle, arose from decaying bodies from "*some seminal particles undiscernedly lurking in some part of the destroyed body ... excited and assisted by a genial and cherishing heat so to act upon the fit and obsequious matter, wherein it was harboured, as to organize and fashion that disposed matter according to the exigencies of its own nature.*"

Athanasius Kircher (1602-1680), a Jesuit priest, linked spontaneous generation with the plague. In a manuscript written in 1658, *On Origin, Causes and Behavior of Plague*, Kircher included, among other possible causes, non-living corpuscles in putrefied matter, which under the "*influence of ambient heat and in proportion to the degree of the infectious decomposition, produce an offspring of innumerable imperceptible worms.*" These worms, which he had seen using a "*very delicate*" microscope, were small enough to infect porous matter or to enter the body by breathing or by contact with fingers or other forms of contact.

Incredibly enough, Kircher managed to avoid church censoring even though he was an affirmed believer in the historical Hermes, dating him to the time of Abraham. Perhaps he was saved by the fact that he used Hermes not to promote alchemy but instead to incorporate his writings as part of his historical studies of Egyptian hieroglyphics and theology, even to the point of including lists of astral imagery found in Hermetic texts.

Germs of Contagion - The Path Least Taken

Suppose, for example, that the circumambient air carries certain seeds of plague, and that the bodies which share (breathe) it, some are full of residues which are soon to become putrefied in themselves, while others are clean and

---

[17] When fermental odor settles upon a part of the body it gives rise to toxic symptoms that can only be driven out by a beneficial odor. This is another reason that herbs and plants occupied a central place in van Helmont's therapeutic methods.

free of such residues. Assume also that in the former there is a general blockage of their pores ....The others ... a wholesome transpiration through pores that are neither blocked nor constricted ... which of these bodies is most likely to be affected by the rotting air they inspire? (Galen)

That the air contained invisible seeds and that these seeds might cause disease is an ancient idea, as suggested in this text of Galen. However, Galen paid hardly any attention to it, probably because it did not alter his conception of the internal disease process and the means whereby the physician might bring about a cure. Galen's greater concern, as was that of Hippocrates, was to determine the peculiar nature of each individual that made them prone to illness, and to seek remedies, including diet, which would correct humoral imbalance.

As seen earlier, both Hippocrates and Galen favored bad air as a cause of epidemics. From his own experience, Galen had traced bad air to unburied corpses on the battlefield, mephitic vapors emerging from the earth's depths, marshes and stagnant pools, and the like. There was no reason to imagine the existence of invisible seeds or germs to explain the action of bad air.

Thinking on this matter continued throughout the Middle Ages, especially in the philosophical debate concerning causation and, in particular, action at a distance. Although several contemporary writers addressed these questions, the work of Girolamo Fracastoro (1478-1553) is generally credited to be the most evolved and thorough statement of its time and thus deserving greater attention.

Fracastoro was a physician who practiced in Verona until 1534 when he retired to devote himself to his writings. His poem, *Syphilis or the French Sickness*, modeled on Virgil's *Georgics*, describes the terrible disease syphilis, as well as it gave it its modern name. The poem tells the adventures of a rich and beautiful shepherd Syphilus who insulted Apollo and was punished with a terrible disease that stripped his limbs of flesh, made his teeth fall out and his breath rotten smelling, and reduced his voice to a whisper. Much of Fracastoro's immediate fame derived from the success with which this long epic poem was greeted.

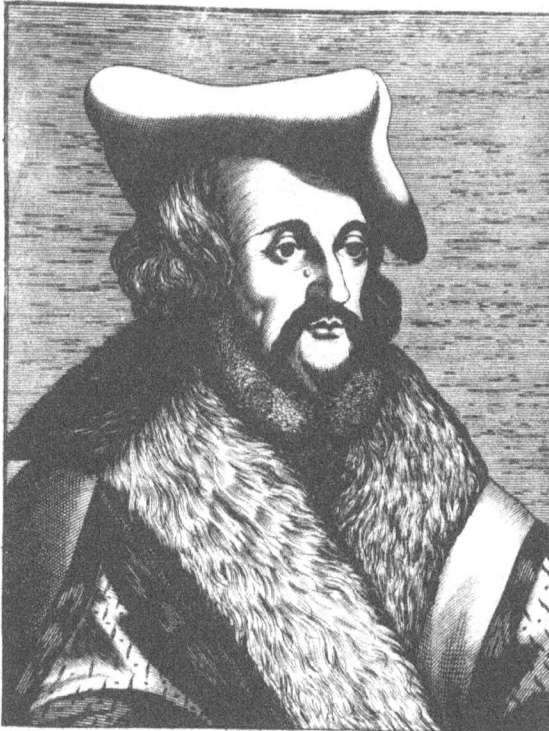

HIERONYMVS   FRACASTORIVS
De Larmessin scul.

Fracastoro's *Contagion, Contagious Diseases and their Treatment* appeared in 1546. He worked on this text for 16 years before its publication, writing *"not as a poet, but as a doctor."* It is this work that particularly concerns us, since in it he developed a theory of contagion based primarily on 'seminaria' or germs/seeds of disease. Although this theory is highly speculative, his practical observations concerning contagious diseases allowed him to be the first to describe typhus as a disease distinct from plague, and also to re-establish tuberculosis (phthisis), largely neglected since Hippocrates' time, as an infectious disease.

Fracastoro devoted some 30 pages of his book to the subject of contagion, in which he addressed such subjects as - What is Contagion? The Fundamental Differences in Contagions; How the Germs of Contagions are Carried to a Distant Object and in a Circle; and Is Every Contagion a Kind of Putrefaction? His style of approaching the subject is a highly logical one, in which arguments are developed by analogy and ancient and current beliefs are selectively used. So smooth and continuous is his delivery and so coherent the end product that it is hard to find any place where it can easily be countered.

"Contagion is an infection that passes from one thing to another." This, as Fracastoro informs us on the opening page, follows from its name. A poison is an infection but not a contagion since only the poisoned party is affected; it does not spread to anyone else. A house that catches fire from the burning of a neighboring house is *"certainly not"* a contagion, since the whole house is involved all at once. Fracastoro allows the term contagion only to apply to an infection that *"originates in very small imperceptible particles."*

There are three *"fundamentally different types of contagion - the first infects by direct contact only; the second does the same, but in addition leaves fomites, and this contagion may spread by means of fomites, for instance scabies, phthisis ... thirdly, there is a kind of contagion which is transmitted not only by direct contact or by fomites as intermediary, but also infects at a distance; for example, pestilent fevers, phthisis ..."* By fomites he meant *"clothes, wooden objects, and things of that sort, which though not themselves corrupted can, nevertheless, preserve the original germs of the contagion and infect by means of these."*[18] The first and third types had long been familiar, but he may have been the first to introduce fomites.

Contagion that infects by contact only is the easiest of the three types to describe, since it is analogous to contagion in fruits - *"as when grape infects grape, or apple infects apple."* Infection derives from *"touch"* by means of which putrefaction is passed from one fruit to the next. Putrefaction is *"a sort of dissolution of a combination due to evaporation of the innate warmth and moisture."* The heat that caused the putrefaction in the first fruit came *"either from the air or some other source."* The dissolved particles from the first fruit can act on the second fruit independently as well as in combination. Two combinations are possible, either *"hot and dry"* or *"hot and moist."* Only the latter are *"apt to produce putrefaction,"* while the former are more *"apt to burn."* The particles that cause putrefaction are called *"Germs of Contagion."*

Contagion that infects by fomites does not occur along the lines of direct contact, since fomites, i.e. germ carrying objects, may last for years, as witness smells that emit from soot-covered walls, while *"particles that evaporate from putrefying bodies never seem to have the power to last as long as that."* The particles that adhere to fomites must be ones that are both fine and volatile individually but strong and resistant in combination. Their fineness and volatility allows them to penetrate the pores of certain objects where they remain not *"exposed to the air or to alteration from outside."* Being strong, *"they can hold out against many attacks."* Also, such germs are *"viscous and sticky."* Otherwise they would not stick or they would easily be washed away. Wool, rags, and many kinds of wood are *"well adapted"* to be fomites. Whether

---

[18] The singular of fomites, *fomes*, literally means 'tinder' and derives from theology where it represents the minute portion of original sin left behind after baptism, which when presented with a suitably desirable object, might burst into the fire of concupiscence.

fomites cause infection or not depend upon whether the body touched by the fomites is *"analogous with that originally infected."*

Contagion at a distance is a well-known fact, as indicated in Fracastoro's opening statement:

> *It is well known that pestiferous fevers, phthisis and many other diseases infect those who live with the sufferer, even though there is no actual contact. It is far from certain what is the nature of these diseases, and how the taint is propagated. We must therefore study these problems with the greatest care, since of this sort are the majority of the diseases that we are investigating.*

Fracastoro begins by examining certain properties and qualities of matter and things, along the lines of Aristotle and Hippocrates. Material qualities are contrasted with 'spiritual' ones. The former include *"hot, cold, moist, dry; light, smell, taste and sound,"* while the latter *"are the manifestations and images of material qualities ... for instance 'luminousness' is the spiritual quality of light."* Hot, cold, moist and dry are *"primary"* and *"generate and alter everything."* Light, taste, smell and sound are *"secondary"* and, while not interacting with each other, they *"do nevertheless arouse the senses, thought only by the mediation of the qualities called spiritual."*

Having established these 'facts', Fracastoro goes on to challenge those who invoke occult properties, e.g. evil spirits and the devil, to explain by what qualities, material or spiritual, contagions are produced. It must be one or the other. If material, it must be one that is known, since *"it is quite impossible ... to invent some unknown kind of quality which is not heat, moisture, or dryness."* Spiritual factors are ruled out because these *"can only last just so long as there is present the source whence they flowed, except indeed when they arise in the intellect."* Since fomites endure for a long time, to invoke spiritual qualities, is to *"resort to the unnecessary and assign an incongruous cause."* He concludes this section by indicating that *"in these contagions, not only putrefaction must be produced, but from the original germs other germs must be begotten and propagated that are similar to those former germs both in their nature and combination ..."*

Fracastoro then establishes that contagion at a distance involves the passage of germs through the air from one person to another. Next, three methods are identified whereby these germs might penetrate the body - propagation in the *"neighboring humors"*; attraction, *"partly through the breath by inspiration, partly by dilatation of the blood-vessels"*; and entry into the small and narrow blood-vessels which are near the periphery, from where they can easily diffuse to the larger blood-vessels, "*where there is greater heat, and thence it is carried even to the heart, unless there be some obstacle.*"

Those germs that adhere to the "*neighboring humors*" will "*generate and propagate others, until the whole mass and bulk of humors is infected by them.*" Those germs that enter by inspiration "*do not retire as easily by expiration ... for they adhere closely to the humors and organs, and some even to the spirits, which retreat from the image of their contrary, and carry their enemy with them even to the heart.*" Germs do not attack the heart, as such, since they neither possess "*cognition*" nor "*will.*"

By drawing analogies with wine that putrefies and rabid dogs that are attacked by a sort of fever, Fracastoro concludes that every contagion is a putrefaction. However, he admits of many cases where there is "*great putrefaction but no contagion.*" For example, there are fevers that are very inflammatory but because they "*have a dry composition ... the particles that evaporate from them cannot be the germs of contagion in something else.*" On the other hand, "*fevers that have a foul and confined putrefaction produce germs suitable for conveying contagions.*"

Fracastoro recognized the specificity of diseases, a concept that is central to the development of the microbial basis of diseases, as discussed in Chapter VI. Observing that certain pests attack trees and crops but not animals, and vice versa, he reasons that each contagion differs with respect to which humors they affect and to what degree they are "*fatal to the spirits.*" In his more detailed consideration of the "*pestilent fevers*" he concludes, contrary to Galen, that the peculiar character of such fevers is not related to the humors affected but primarily to the specific nature of the diseases - "*The principles of contagions per se are the germs themselves.*"

Had Fracastoro stopped at this point, his description of contagion would have been complete and recognizably 'modern'. Instead, he went on to add that diseases were caused by germs that could "*arise first in us,*" i.e. a form of spontaneous generation, and to profess his belief that stars and planets influenced the onset of epidemics. Both of these points, as we have seen earlier, were commonly accepted well into the 17th century. That he was a skilled astronomer provides further evidence of the importance he gave to astral influences.

Phthisis and pestiferous fevers are examples given of diseases whose germs first arise inside the body. This can happen because "*in us and our humors there is nothing to prevent the production of putrefactions that are both foul and confined, from which develop germs that are both viscous and have a strong combination."* Once *"engendered in an individual, and from the general disposition of the atmosphere, they transfer the contagion to another."* While the air *"is the most potent cause"* of contagions which come from without, *"they may also arise from water, marshes and other sources."*

The *"heavenly bodies"* do not produce contagion directly. They, however, *"may of themselves become heated, and this increase of heat results in the rise of a great mass of vapors from the waters and the earth; these vapors presently may produce various and diverse kinds of corruption, some new, some familiar to us, some unusually severe, according to the different constitutions of those heavenly bodies."* The most serious effects are those *"in which several of the planets are in conjunction; especially under the influence of certain of those important stars that are called 'fixed'."*

The air can provide signs of contagion of its own, such as *"falling stars, comets, fiery beams (aurora), tempest-flares and the like, which indicate that putrefaction is occurring around the earth. For all these arise from an unctuous (oily) and viscous fomites."* Moreover, there are conditions of the *"lower atmosphere"* to observe, e.g.

> *the danger when the south winds blow strong and for a long period; or when one sees abnormal mists hanging over a certain region; or finally, if a brownish and dusty sort of atmosphere has for a long time made the sun look gloomy.*

> *But one needs especially to be on one's guard when one observes that certain winds are blowing from a quarter where the plague prevails; and one should not merely fear, but flee, when objects placed in the open air, such as provisions, linen and the like, contract a kind of decay and mildew. But the waters too give their own signs, when rivers overflow, and the inundations last for a long time, and then leave behind them marshy and muddy places; also when the sea discharges on to its shores many dead fish.*

The work of Fracastoro provides a rich and unique introduction to the multiple ways that different kinds of contagion were thought to arise, including germ seeds. Nevertheless, the idea of germs failed to gain any following; instead, the traditional Hippocratic-Galenic ideas concerning noxious air and receptive bodies prevailed. Fracastoro's medical colleagues dismissed his germ idea just like he had dismissed 'spiritual qualities'. Germs were superfluous and unnecessary since they added yet another element to an already long list of possible causes without adding any new understanding to the disease-causation process itself.[19] Also, he was found to be wrong in certain of his conclusions. For example, his categorical statement that *"putrefaction must be produced"* by contagious diseases was clearly contrary to the many deaths observed during epidemics involving no bodily putrefaction.

On the Epidemic Constitution of the Atmosphere

It might be worth while to consider, whether these coalitions of differing sorts of steams in the air, and the changes resulting thence of their particular precedent quantities, may not assist us to investigate the causes of divers sudden clouds and mists, and some other meteorological phaenomena, and also of divers changes that happen in the air, in reference to the coming in and ceasing of several either epidemical, or contagious diseases, and particularly the plague, that seems to depend upon some occult temperature and alterations of the air, which may be copiously impregnated by the differing subterraneal (not to add here, sidereal) effluviums, that not unfrequently ascend into it, or otherwise invade it, with pestiferous, or other morbifick corpuscles. (Boyle)

The French court physician, Guillaume de Baillou (1538-1616), is credited for having resurrected the ancient Hippocratic idea of the epidemic constitution of the atmosphere. He was a skillful physician, a brilliant teacher, and an acute observer. He insisted upon the study of patients, of nature, and of disease pictures, and was a vehement champion of the methods of Hippocrates. He participated in post-mortem examinations, including those of Jeanne d'Albret, the Queen of Navarre, and Charles IX of France. He differentiated between rheumatism and gout, as Hippocrates had done. He described in a striking manner plague, diphtheria, rheumatic fever and whooping cough, the latter being the first description of that disease. His clinical case histories sometimes included the influence of environmental and hereditary factors.

---

[19] To indicate just how hard it is to understand how physicians differed in their notions of disease-causing agents, Girolamo Mercuriale, a Venician physician, argued that all agreed on the origin of plague but that they were using different terminology. He took the miasmas of Hippocrates, the atoms of Democritus, and the seeds of Lucretius all to be the 'same'!

Plague Legends

Taking Hippocrates as his model, Baillou advocated the idea that only a study of the weather prevailing immediately before or during the occurrence of an outbreak of disease can guide proper treatment. However, he recorded little meteorological detail; instead, he drew rather general conclusions such as - the wet spring of 1571 was one in which many people had colds, pleurisy, and sore throats, and the hot summer of 1578 was followed by an epidemic of whooping cough.

He believed that the heavenly bodies exert an influence on humans, having witnessed directly the convulsions, deliriums and disturbances caused by the solar eclipse in December 1573. He found *"something divine"* about the south wind that prevailed during the winter of 1576, which, however, was only able to act due to a particular disposition of the bodily organs. On two occasions he used the term 'germs' in the general sense of disease origin or cause. In one he states that mercury possesses a protective quality against all germs' of corruption, because it is the 'germ' of all the metals.

Baillou's epidemiological text *On Epidemic and Ephemeral Diseases*, in which he described his theories and findings, did not get published until 1640. There is some evidence that Sydenham was familiar with this work.

Boyle, as indicated in the quote above, also believed in the role of the atmosphere in the origin of disease. His interest in the atmosphere included efforts to conceptualise the physical makeup of air and to understand the role of air as a medium of transport for effluvial particles that sloughed off from earthly matter. He allowed for the possibility that air could alter the constitution of some of these particles, even going so far as to express the possibility that 'new diseases' might arise from *"some yet unobserved commerce between the earth and other mundane globes."* He encouraged detailed meteorological studies using recently developed instruments to measure temperature, atmospheric pressure, wind velocity, humidity, and rainfall for comparative analyses of disease trends in different areas.[20]

As noted earlier, Sydenham was a close friend of Boyle. It was on Boyle's *"persuasion and recommendation"* that Sydenham began the clinical study of

---

[20] Boyle's research concerning the *"hidden qualities of air"* and the fact that air was needed to keep *"flame and fire alive,"* led him to *"suspect that there may be dispersed through the rest of the atmosphere some odd substance, either of a solar, or astral, or some other exotic nature..."* Some 100 years later oxygen was shown to be the substance needed to keep flames *"alive"* but no longer was its origin conceived to be *"exotic."*

London's epidemics. Following fourteen years of study he recognized five periods that were characterized by a particular 'epidemic constitution' or disposition of the atmosphere. But as hard as he tried, he could not correlate atmospheric conditions with the different epidemic diseases present. He was forced to conclude instead that - "*Years that coincide in appreciable atmospheric characters differ in their diseases and vice versa.*"

This led him at first to define an epidemic in the following rather unsatisfactory manner:

Some (acute diseases) are engendered through occult and inexplicable changes in the atmosphere. These taint the human body but they depend upon the peculiar crases of our blood and humours only so far as these occult atmospheric influences have made an impression on them. Such maladies continue their devastation during the continuance of the mysterious atmospheric constitution but not longer. These diseases are called epidemics.

In time, however, Sydenham turned more and more towards Boyle's morbific particles and "*subterraneal effluviums.*" By 1683, Sydenham came to explain epidemics as follows:

Whether the inward bowels of the earth undergo various changes by the vapours which exhale therefrom so that the air is tainted, or whether the atmosphere be changed by some alterations induced by some peculiar conjunction of any of the heavenly bodies, it is a truth that at particular times the air is stuffed full of particles which are hostile to the economy of the human body...At these times whenever we draw in with our breath such noxious and unnatural miasmata, mix them with our blood, and fall into such epidemic diseases as they are apt to engender, Nature calls in fever as her usual instrument for expelling from the blood any hostile materials that may lurk in it. Such diseases are usually called epidemic.

Sydenham's description of an epidemic of coughs in the winter of 1679 (influenza) illustrates well both his conception of an acute disease brought about by external "*particles*" entering the body and how the body reacts to fend off the attack. He conceived the epidemic's cause as being due to the wetter-than-usual month of October which led to the blood drinking in an "*abundance of crude, watery particles.*" When the first cold came, "*perspiration was stopt,*" and Nature endeavored to expel these particles "*by means of a cough, through the branches of the pulmonary artery, or, as some will have it, through the glands of the windpipe.*"

Plague Legends

Sydenham distinguished two broad groups of epidemics, one arising in the spring (vernal) and the other in the fall (autumnal). The former included measles and *"vernal tertians"* and the latter - plague, smallpox, autumnal dysenteries, tertians and quartans. However, he gave priority to the epidemic constitution prevailing in any given year over the identification of specific disease epidemics. This allowed him to conclude that *"in whatever years these several species (of diseases) prevail at one and the same time, the symptoms wherewith they come on are alike in all."* He also believed that one epidemic tended to expel another. His inability to judge from measurable atmospheric conditions which disease was present forced him to take a 'wait and see' attitude when new fevers arose before deciding upon the line of therapy to follow.

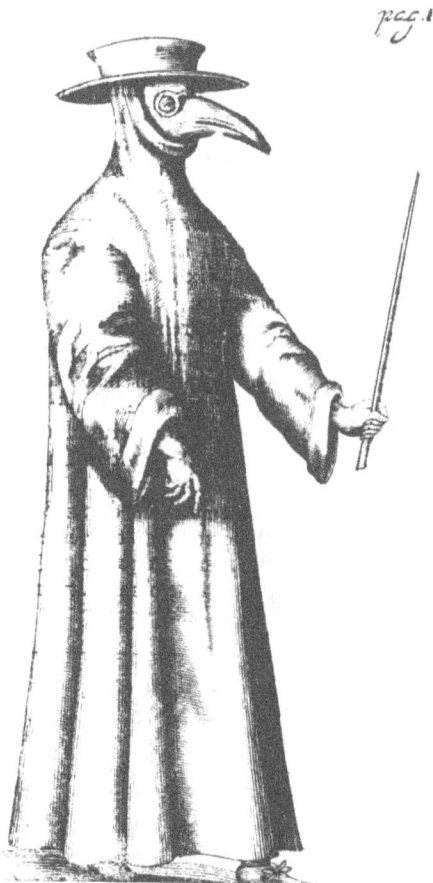

fig.1

Sydenham prudently fled London with his wife and young family when the plague broke out, joining the many others who had the chance. Because of his later fame, it is of interest to note that he later claimed that it was produced by the receiving of *"effluvia, or seminium, from an infected person."*[21] Then the *"whole air of that tract of land is quickly infected with the plague, by means of the breath of the disease, and the steam or vapor arising from the dead bodies, so as to render the way of propagating this dreadful disease by infection entirely unnecessary …"*

Although some two hundred years had passed from the time that Ficino had written his plague treatise, the basic ingredients had remained more or less the same, resembling much that could be traced all the way back to Hippocrates. Ficino wrote of *"earth poisons"* while Sydenham relied on

---

[21] Although it did not become part of his analytic considerations, Sydenham did acknowledge that plague was *"the scourge for the enormity of our sins."*

"*vapours*" exhaled from "*the bowels of the earth.*" Both imagined that the conjunction of heavenly bodies might be one of the necessary conditions to trigger the creation of "*pestilential air.*" Both, too, saw the importance of the body being pre-disposed to illness. Finally, both invoked the image of putrefying humors to explain the onset of fever and both portrayed fever as the means whereby the body seeks to fight off disease. This, by the way, is consistent with the modern view of fever.

* * * * *

As the more conservative religious thinking gained command, astrology and Hermeticism, at least as practiced and believed in by physicians, slowly died out. Alchemy, as well, no longer formed part of the scientific mainstream. Nevertheless, its remnants could still be found among the beliefs of leading scientists at the end of the 17th century. Isaac Newton (1642-1727), for example, practiced alchemy and expressed interest in the ideas of the Rosicrucians and the writings of Fludd. He and Boyle shared alchemical information, although he was far more secretive than Boyle was in letting others know of his interest and work in alchemy. In one of his alchemical notes he quotes Hermes Trismegistus as saying - "*I had this art and science by the sole inspiration of God who has vouchsafed to reveal it to his servant.*" It is probably through Fludd's writings that he learned of Hermes Trismegistus. In fact, it may have been the Hermetic ideas that he found there that inspired the sweeping hypothesis of gravitational attraction, a universal force operating through empty space.

God's hand remained present but in an ever-diminishing manner, as science developed and an ever-increasing number of natural phenomena were placed on a sound empirical basis.

What had not been disposed of was the Hippocratic 'epidemic constitution of the atmosphere'. Instead, by the beginning of the 18th century, the reasons whereby the atmosphere could become 'pestilential' had grown, having accumulated an extraordinarily rich assortment of ideas, ideas that stemmed from logical observations as much as from philosophical musings on the nature of the universe. That disease might be caused by 'germ' particles was an ever-present but not seriously considered idea.

While it proved difficult to ascertain it scientifically, the 'epidemic atmosphere' gained the upper hand as an explanatory feature in all major disease outbreaks; it fitted comfortably all disease-causation theories. However, when it came to what steps to be taken to prevent or control outbreaks, important differences arose, especially as regards whether to quarantine or not. At issue was precisely how it was believed the atmosphere gained its epidemic qualities, as discussed further in Chapters V and VI. Deciding upon the utility of quarantine, in particular, grew even more problematic after the new diseases of yellow fever and cholera appeared. Only with the recognition of the essential role of germs, as described in Chapter VI, could (nearly) all facts concerning epidemics be explained.

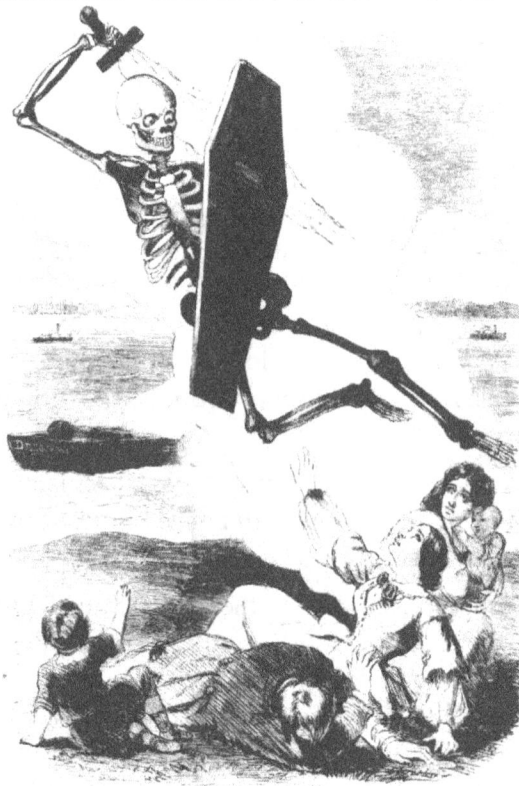

THE QUARANTINE QUESTION.

DEATH, RISING FROM THE QUARANTINE SCOW, AND SCATTERING PESTILENCE AMONG THE PEOPLE.

PART II - DISEASE PROFILES

IV

Disease Profiles

For uncovering hidden diseases is not like recognizing colors. With colors the observer sees black, green, blue and so on; but if they had a curtain in front of them he would not know them; to see through a curtain would required spectacles such as never were. What the eyes tell may be diagnosed at once but it is useless to diagnose that which is hidden from sight, treating it as though it were plainly visible. (Paracelsus)

Paracelsus believed in disease specificity, that is, that diseases were real objects that can be examined and classified like any other object. Van Helmont imagined classifying diseases according to their specific idea or image (creative 'seed'). This specificity would be recognized by specific organ changes, independent of the human body in which each organ was located. However, he did not have the means to demonstrate that idea; it would only be in the 18th century that the necessary tools and skills would be available to diagnose disease according to internal changes in the body.

Sydenham, on the other hand, recognized the existence of specific diseases in the visible symptoms of his patients:

He who observes attentively the order, the time, the hour at which the attack of quart fever begins, the phenomena of shivering, of heat, in a word all the symptoms proper to it, will have as many reasons to believe that this disease is a species as he has to believe that a plant constitutes a species because it grows, flowers, and dies always in the same way.

Fever occupied an important place in his studies and reflections. Many, if not most, of the common diseases present in 17th century England had fever as one of the presenting symptoms. While smallpox and measles were readily identified by their skin eruptions, there were many other febrile diseases that were not so easily distinguishable, e.g. typhoid, typhus, influenza, tuberculosis, and malaria.

Classifiers did not know how many diseases existed. Today, as reflected by the relatively small number of diseases described in this chapter, the total number of diseases recognized is far less than, for example, the 2400 disease 'species' identified in 1762 by François Boissier de Sauvages (1706-67), professor of medicine at Montpellier. That he thought such a large number of diseases existed is not surprising when it is realized that factors such as force and speed of the pulse, intensity of pain, and violence of cough were used to distinguish one from another. It should be noted, as well, that Boissier de Sauvages and his fellow classifiers did not concern themselves with the presence of a disease in an organ, since they believed that disease could travel from one point in the body to another. Others, for example the early neurologist Robert Whytt (1714-66), still believed that the place and working of the human 'soul' played an important part in disease physiology, despite Descartes' efforts to argue the contrary.

Plague

History[22]

Although the Bible and other ancient texts mention 'plague', it is generally held that the true plague did not arrive in Europe until it burst upon the Mediterranean world in AD 542. It spread to Ireland and England but did not enter northern Europe at that time. After several centuries of respite, it returned to Europe in 1347. The Black Death, as it quickly came to be known, was particularly devastating. This time it spread north and before the year's end was in Germany and England. When it was over, at least 25 million had perished in Europe alone, or one-fourth to one-third of its population.

When it first arrived in 1347, the population was entirely susceptible, which accounts for the horrifying death tolls. Once it swept across the Continent, it remained endemic, smoldering until enough non-immunes were present to allow it to flare-up again. This pattern continued for several centuries. The last major outbreak in England was London's plague in 1665. The last major epidemics in Europe occurred in Marseilles in 1720 and in Moscow in 1771. There would still be one small outbreak in Essex, England in 1909, but for now it seems that it has died out from Europe for good. The brown or sewer rat, which replaced the black rat, is much less dangerous as a transmitter of plague, thus largely accounting for plagues' disappearance from Europe. Today, plague is mostly confined to foci in Africa, America and Asia.

---

[22] *History* covers epidemic outbreaks from earliest recorded times through the 19th century, with an occasional mention of relevant 20th century events.

Etiology

Plague is caused by a bacterium, *Yersina pestis*, which is a natural parasite of small wild animals, especially rodents, and is transmitted by fleas. Normally, plague is not a disease of human beings. Under usual circumstances, the bacterium rests in wild animal populations, carried from animal to animal by fleas. In an infected animal, the bacteria are present in the blood where it passes into the flea's stomach with its meal. Here plague bacilli multiply and are ready to be passed over to an uninfected animal when the flea next bites.

The black rat better supports fleas that are ready to bite man as well as rats. Black rats reached Europe from India with the returning Crusaders; this factor explains plague's more extensive spread the second time around. As the Black Death developed, rat-to-human transmission was largely replaced by human-to-human, either by way of fleas, or directly through the air when the disease took the pneumonic form. Evidence suggests that during the winter of 1347-48, the pneumonic form was dominant, while in the summer that followed, nearly all victims contracted the bubonic form. The difference between the two forms is a function of how severe the infection is. Only in severe infections do the bacilli reach the lymph glands where they cause inflammation and swelling, giving rise to buboes from which bubonic plague is named. Pneumonic plague, as the name implies, is mostly confined to an infection of the lungs.

Clinical course

During the 1656-57 epidemic in Rome, the symptoms of plague were reported as follows:

> *Onset is marked with very high temperature, very severe headache, bilious vomiting, sleepiness, occasional diarrhea, and cloudy, dark urine. Quite often delirium supervened on the 2nd day. In many patients buboes and carbuncles appeared with the first attack of temperature. Other and more numerous patients suffered from such a mild temperature that they did not seem to run any temperature at all, but they experienced such severe prostration and such a loss of all natural vital and animal faculties that none reached the 3rd day, and yet they showed no exterior signs or petechiae (rash) on their bodies.*

Plague was differentiated from other disease of the time by the buboes under the armpit and in the groin and the true carbuncles. Other signs, e.g. high temperature, the petechiae, large spots on the skin, mental dullness and headache, delirium, sleepiness, vomiting and cloudy urine, were symptoms common to a number of other diseases.

Montaigne, at the end of the 16th century, observed that during a raging epidemic:

> *All illnesses are then taken to be the plague: no time is allowed to probe them. And (best of all!) according to the rules of the Art, every time you are exposed to risk, you spend your quarantine in an ecstatic dread of that illness; your imagination meanwhile has its own way of agitating you, making your very health sweat with fever... It is not the worst of deaths: it is normally short, marked by numbness and lack of pain, comforted by being shared with many, without ritual and without a crowd of mourners.*

Smallpox

History

Unmistakable descriptions of smallpox first appeared in the 4th century AD in China. The earliest records of it in Europe date in the 7th century from the Mediterranean area. However, some historians have suggested that the 'Plague of Athens' that occurred in 430 BC may have been smallpox. That outbreak lasted for over 2 years, totally devastating the Athenian army.

Advancing and retreating armies in the Middle Ages spread the disease so that by the latter half of the 10th century it was common in most of the Arab-controlled areas of Europe. The Crusades of the 11th and 12th centuries further spread the disease in Europe and caused numerous severe epidemics. For example, Iceland lost 20,000 of its total population of about 70,000 in 1241. By the 15th century smallpox had become endemic in many parts of Europe, but not as severe as it then became in the 17th and 18th centuries, when it succeeded plague, leprosy and syphilis as the continent's foremost pestilence.

Smallpox reached England in the early decades of the 17th century. European explorers and colonists introduced smallpox into South and North America from the 16th century onwards. The rapid and fatal course of the disease among indigenous peoples, especially in the Americas, played an important part in helping Europeans conquer new territories. By the mid-18th century smallpox was a major endemic disease throughout the world except in Australia and in several small islands.

Etiology

Smallpox is caused by two strains of virus named *Variola major* and *minor*; the latter is responsible for a milder form of the disease.[23] The virus has only been found in humans and can persist in populations only if enough susceptible humans are constantly available to maintain a continuous chain of infection. Smallpox scabs can retain infectivity at room temperatures for several years; under tropical conditions, the virus generally does not survive in the scab for more than 16 weeks.

Clinical course

Up until the end of the 19th century, smallpox was regarded as a distinct disease of great severity and high case-fatality rate. Subsequently outbreaks were seen with relatively low case fatality rates (1% or less), suggesting the presence of different strains of the virus.

Rhazes (860-932), a celebrated physician known as the Arabian Hippocrates, left this description of those symptoms that precede the eruption of the smallpox:

> *The eruption of the smallpox is preceded by a continued fever, pain in the back, itching in the nose, and terrors in sleep. These are the more peculiar symptoms of its approach, especially a pain in the back, with fever; then also a pricking which the patient feels all over his body; a fullness of the face, which at times goes and comes; an inflamed color, and vehement redness in both the cheeks; a redness of both the eyes; a heaviness of the whole body; great uneasiness, the symptoms of which are stretching and yawning; a pain in the throat and chest, with a slight difficulty in breathing, and cough; a dryness of the mouth, thick spittle, and hoarseness of the voice; pain and heaviness of the head; inquietude, distress of the mind, nausea, and anxiety; heat of the whole body, an inflamed color, and shining redness, and especially an intense redness of the gums.*

A body rash appears shortly after the onset of fever. Several days after the onset of the rash, skin eruptions begin, increasing in severity over time.

---

[23] Following a global eradication campaign conducted by the World Health Organisation, the world's last naturally occurring case of smallpox was recorded in October 1977. However, there still remain several stockpiles of the live virus that have not as yet been destroyed.

Scabbing begins during the second week, when in most fatal cases, death occurs. Among survivors, the scabs separate by the 4th week.

Tuberculosis

History

Tuberculosis is one of the most ancient of diseases and has been described by many writers, including Hippocrates. The Greek word 'phthisis' was adopted and used to describe wasting diseases of the chest. Later, other terms were added to designate it, such as 'consumption' and 'hectic fever'. The generic name 'tuberculosis' itself derives from the tubercles found in consumptive cases upon autopsy and seems first to have been used around 1840. Also appearing in the 19th century was the designation 'White Plague'.

Not killing in an explosive manner like the true plague, tuberculosis insidiously invades a community and does its killing slowly but relentlessly, where it has not been controlled. At the end of the 18th century in England, pulmonary tuberculosis was considered by far the most deadly disease. It was the chief cause of death in the United States until 1904.

Since the symptoms of tuberculosis overlap those of many other chronic diseases, it has proved impossible to develop any accurate picture of its prevalence before recent times. Only when its obvious manifestations have been recorded can there be any certainty of its presence. One such clue is swollen nodes, particularly those of the neck. The expression 'scrofulous' was used to describe these nodes, and from the 5th up until the late 18th century, it was believed in France that if the king at the time of his anointment were to touch the swollen glands the individuals would be cured. English kings claimed this power as well in the 11th century. With this belief, tuberculosis (scrofula) gained yet another name, that of the 'King's Evil'. William Shakespeare (1564-1616), in *Macbeth*, describes the touch as follows:

> *... strangely-visited people*
> *All swol'n and ulcerous, pitiful to the eye,*
> *The mere despair of surgery, he cures,*
> *Hanging a golden stamp about their necks,*
> *Put on with holy prayers; and 'tis spoken,*
> *To the succeeding royalty he leaves*
> *The healing benediction ...*

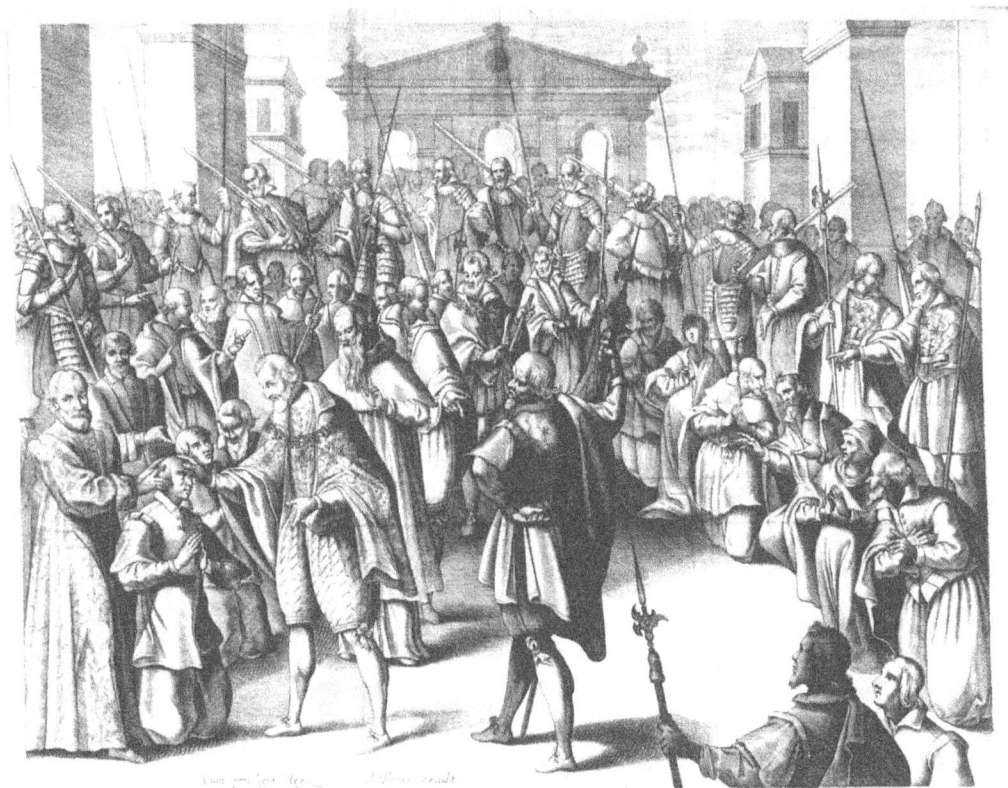

Etiology

Tuberculosis is caused by a bacillus that bears its name, *Mycobacterium tuberculosis*. It spreads easily being transmitted by coughing or sneezing. Contaminated minute droplets sometimes contain hundreds of tubercle bacilli and may float in the air for hours.

Clinical course

The principle site of tuberculosis is the lung. Ordinarily pulmonary tuberculosis is a chronic disease, although it may on occasion be 'fulminating', in which case extensive destruction of the lung tissue takes place in a few months. In its chronic form it waxes and wanes with long periods of apparent remission followed by periods of exacerbation.

Tuberculosis causes little discomfort during its initial stages and thus may remain unnoticed by the patient for some time. By the time medical attention is sought, the disease usually is already in a very advanced form. Hippocrates' description of the symptoms of tuberculosis is as follows:

> *fevers accompanied by rigors, of the continual type, acute, having no complete intermissions, but of the forms of semi-tertians, being milder the one day and the next having an exacerbation, and increasing in violence; constant sweats, but not diffused over the whole body; extremities very cold, and warmed with difficulty; bowels disordered, with bilious, scanty, unmixed, thin, and pungent, and frequent dejections. The urine was thin, colorless, unconcocted, or thick, with a deficient sediment, not settling favorably, but casting down a crude and unseasonable sediment. Sputa small, dense, concocted, but brought up rarely and with difficulty; and in those who encountered the most violent symptoms there was no concoction at all, but they continued throughout spitting crude matters. Their fauces, in most of them, were painful from the first to last, having redness with inflammation; defluxions thin, small, and acrid; they were soon wasted and became worse, having no appetite for any kind of food throughout; no thirst; most persons delirious when near death.*

John Keats, the English poet, died of tuberculosis in 1821 at the age of 26. His description of tuberculosis written in the spring of 1819 is perhaps the most poignant one of all:

> *Youth grows pale, and spectre thin, and dies*

Diphtheria

History

When Bretonneau (see Chapter VI) sought to find historical evidence showing the presence of diphtheria in ancient times, the earliest reference he could find was in the works of Aretaeus, who in the 2nd century AD described ulcers of the throat that he believed to have come from Egypt and Syria. Aetius, the personal physician of the Emperor Justinian I (483-565), provided one of the best early descriptions of diphtheria (see below). "*Perhaps less from want of occasions for observation than from want of observers*" Bretonneau wrote, "*that we must pass from the fifth to the end of the sixteenth century to find the disease again well described.*"

From that time on diphtheria has "*almost constantly shown itself in every region of the old or new continent.*" At first, it continued for some time in Spain in the form of murderous epidemics. Because one form of illness frequently led to suffocation, the Spaniards called it *morbres suffocares* or the *garrotillo*, garrotes being the sticks used to tighten ropes around the necks of criminals until they strangled to death. So many children died of the disease in 1613 that the year became known in Spanish history as 'the year of the *garrotillo*'.

From Spain it went to Italy and towards the middle of the 18th century epidemics appeared in England, France, Sweden and in America, particularly in New York and Philadelphia. In Italy and Sicily the affliction was known as the 'gullet disease'. John Fothergill published a description of *"the soar throat attended with ulcers"* in 1748, following various outbreaks in London during the previous decade. In 1765, an Edinburgh doctor, believing it to be totally new disease, called it the 'croup', a term which became widely accepted both in England and elsewhere. Samuel Bard seems to be the first American to have described it in his 1771 *An Enquiry into the Nature, Cause, and Cure, of the Angina Suffocativa, &C.* All described the terrible nature of this disease. Writing in 1821, Bretonneau was aware that diphtheria might have been the cause of death of *"the celebrated Washington"* in 1799.

Few cases appeared in England from the late 1820s to the late 1850s but then in 1858 there was a sudden widespread appearance of severe diphtheria there that soon spread to almost every part of the world. Even Australia was infected before the end of the year.

Etiology

Diphtheria is caused by the bacterium *Corynebacterium diphtheriae* and is spread by coughing or sneezing or through contact with skin infections.[24] The bacterium does not invade, but produces surface necrosis in the airways, leading to the formation of a fibrinous pseudo-membrane packed with toxin-generating organisms. It is the toxin that causes destruction and damage throughout the body, including the tonsils, upper respiratory tract, the heart and central nervous system. Like tuberculosis and typhoid, diphtheria can be spread by carriers of the bacillus who are otherwise healthy.

---

[24] Wood tells the story of a Warden of St. Francis, who, suffering from a severe inflammation of the throat, complained of foul breath. To make sure that he was not merely imagining the bad odor, he asked a friend to smell the exhalations from his mouth. Shortly thereafter the friend came down with the illness and died of suffocation on the fourth day. Cortesius (in 1625) who recorded this case, wrote *"from this instance, I have come to the conclusion that the disease is more or less contagious."*

Clinical course

Aretaeus called it the *"pestilential lesions of the tonsils."* Indicating that these lesions occur most frequently in children, he described its clinical course as follows:

> *Usually in children the evils known as aphthae (ulcers) develop. These are white, like blotches; some are ashen in color or like eschars from the cautery. The patient suffers from a dryness of the gullet and frequent attacks of choking ... A spreading sore supervenes in the region afflicted ... In some cases the uvula is eaten up and when the sores have prevailed a long time and deepened, a cicatrix forms over them and the patient's speech becomes rather husky and, in drinking, liquid is diverted upward to the nostrils.*

The complexity of the inflammation process can be judged from some of Bretonneau's observations:

> *The inflammations of the mucous show just as varied characteristics as cutaneous inflammations, whose classification has tested the talent of nosographers. The exudation which accompanies them presents itself some marked differences, sometimes it is a thin fluid, sometimes it consists of mucous variously changed, it is sometimes a coating, which has the whiteness and consistency of caseous material. At other times, it is a membraneous substance closely adherent, or indeed, a membraneous film, simply attached. The degree of thickness, hardness, the force of cohesion, color, the elevation of the tissue effected, the indefinite or limited margin of the inflammation furnish a host of other differences ... co-exist too constantly ... for one not to see here, the relationship of cause and effect.*

Scarlet Fever

History

Scarlet fever is found principally in the temperate zones, rarely in the tropics. Its severity varies over time and place. Since its earliest clear description dates to the early part of the 17th century, scarlet fever's history is mostly unknown. There is no reason, however, to suspect that it was not present much earlier. In the 18th century there were serious epidemics; it seems to have appeared for the first time in America in 1735 as described in Chapter V.

There were fluctuations in the early 19th century, then a steady increase in severity, which culminated in a period of thirty years between 1850 and 1880 when scarlet fever epidemics were frequent and severe in both England and Australia. After 1880 its severity diminished.

Etiology

Scarlet fever may be due to a considerable number of streptococci whose common feature is to produce the toxin responsible for the characteristic scarlet rash. Immunity is mainly to the toxin, not to any specific germ. Thus infection with a mild form produces immunity to potential severe forms of infection.

The disease is spread chiefly by droplet infection but may be disseminated by contaminated dust particles and by contaminated hands, food, drinks and fomites. Contaminated milk, for example, gave rise to several outbreaks recorded in the latter part of the 19th century.

Clinical Course

Sydenham described scarlet fever as follows:

> *Shivers and chills at the commencement; but with no great depression. The whole skin is marked with small, red spots, more frequent, more diffused, and more red than in measles. These last two or three days. They then disappear; leaving the skin covered with branny squamulae, as if powdered with meal.*

Malaria

History

The history of malaria in the western world has been much studied. Nevertheless, some doubts remain concerning which species of malaria were present when and where. For example, although it is clear from the case studies of Hippocrates that he knew malaria, his cases are either that of a tertian or a quartan fever, i.e. *Plasmodium vivax* or *P. malariae* malaria (see etiology below). *P. falciparum* does not seem to have been present. On the other hand, there may have been isolated instances of falciparum malaria, as suggested by Thucydides' description of the autumn illness suffered by the Athenians besieging Syracuse. Galen's observations are more or less identical with those of Hippocrates.

In the late stages of the Roman Empire and throughout the Byzantine period malaria became a much more serious health problem than it had been in early classical times. Increased travel and trade along with 'favorable' ecological changes are thought to have contributed to the spread of the more dangerous malaria-carrying species of anophelines.

Malaria eventually reached nearly all parts of Europe, including as far north as Finland. It waxed and waned over the centuries under the influence of climatic, population, housing and land use factors. Its impact was greatest on the southern parts of the continent but, during the 18th and 19th centuries, it also heavily affected some northern countries.

Dating malaria in the Americas poses a different problem since there is no equivalent to the records left by Hippocrates. Some believe that malaria was not present before the arrival of Europeans and their African slaves; others argue that the use by South American Indians of the bark of the cinchona tree is a clear indication that malaria must have been present before their arrival. An intriguing fact is the presence of human malaria (*P. malariae*) in jungle monkeys and isolated tribes in the Amazon, suggesting the presence of a monkey-human exchange that could date back to pre-Columbian times. Regardless of when and how it got there, by the 18th and 19th century malaria had become one of the major health problems facing new settlers throughout the Americas.

Etiology

Four species of the parasite *Plasmodium* are responsible for human malaria. *P. falciparum* is the most dangerous. Of the other three forms, *P. vivax*, *P. ovale* and *P. malariae*, vivax is by far the most common. Malaria parasites have a complex life cycle involving phases in the stomach of select anopheline mosquitoes, and in the liver and blood of infected humans.

Mosquitoes transmit the parasite to humans as well as ingest it during their blood meals. There are around 60 different anopheline species that can transmit malaria. They differ significantly in a variety of ways, e.g. under what conditions they can best breed and survive, including temperature and humidity; when and where they prefer to bite humans; and how they react to personal protection measures. These differences play an important role in the extent to which the problem is present in any given population.

The incubation period in malaria averages around 12 days for falciparum malaria, 13-15 days for vivax and ovale, and 28-30 days for malariae malaria.

Clinical course

Malaria symptoms include fever, sweating, delirium, lassitude, headache, anorexia, aching of the bones, and vomiting. The cycle of fever is determined by which species is present. *P. falciparum*, *P. vivax* and *P. ovale* give rise to fevers every 48 hours. These are called tertian fevers, i.e. every third day where the count begins on the first fever day. *P. malariae* gives rise to fevers every 72 hours and its fever is called a quartan fever. Mixed infections can give rise to fevers with mixed cycles since each infection is independent of the others.

Cornelius Celsus writing in the 1st century AD described the different malaria fevers as follows:

> *Quartan fevers ... begin commonly with a shuddering; then a heat breaks out; after the paroxysm is over, the patient is well for two days. So that it returns upon the fourth day.*

> *Of tertians ... there are two kinds. One of them both beginning and ending like the quartan; with this difference only, that there is one day's intermission, and it returns upon the third. The other kind is much more fatal, which indeed returns upon the third day, but of the forty-eight hours thirty-six are occupied by the fit (and sometimes either less or more) nor does it entirely cease in the remission; but is only mitigated.*

Cassius, in Shakespeare's Julius Caesar, says of Caesar:

> *He had a fever when he was in Spain,*
> *And, when the fit was on him, I did mark*
> *How he did shake ...*
> *His coward lips did from their colour fly;*
> *And that same eye, ...*
> *Did lose his lustre*

Influenza

History

There is no reason to believe that influenza was not present in ancient times. The earliest case history that some scholars have identified as influenza dates from 1173. Others believe that a definite diagnosis of influenza only dates from 1387. Forty-five serious epidemics of influenza have been recorded from the 15th century on. Most often they have been named after their presumed origins (Russian catarrh, Chinese flu, Scottish rant). That of 1580 may have been the world's first pandemic, i.e. an epidemic of such virulence and mortality as to suggest a major change in the makeup of the influenza virus. North America does not seem to have been reached by any of the European pandemics until that of 1729-30, which did not reach the North American shores until October 1732.

Etiology

Influenza is caused by an airborne virus. Infecting, as it does, the linings of the nose, throat, air passages and lungs, the virus spreads quickly and easily with any form of human contact. There are three types of virus, A, B, and C. Influenza A is responsible for major epidemics and pandemics; it is the only form of the three that is found in animals other than humans. The outbreaks of B tend to be smaller and less severe than those of A. Influenza C does not cause epidemics and causes only mild disease.

Since confirmation of individual disease is rare, the presence of influenza in a population is judged more often than not by its epidemic nature. Other infections might produce similar symptoms, but only influenza results in a sudden appearance of many cases and after a few weeks an equally sudden disappearance of the epidemic. It has been characterized as *"the rogue among epidemic diseases, suddenly cutting loose and sweeping across the world with a speed and a ferocity unequalled by any other disease."*

As noted above, it is the changing nature of the influenza A virus that gives rise to new pandemics. In marked contrast to other viral agents such as polio virus or measles virus, it seems that there is little stability of influenza strains in nature. Like all viral microorganisms, it is a self-replicating agent of disease. The virus invades a host cell and commandeers it to produce hundreds of copies of the viral genetic material, which for the influenza virus takes the form of 8 segments or chromosomes of RNA. These RNA segments encode two glycoproteins which are embedded on the lipid (fat) surface of the virus - hemagglutinin (H) and neuraminidase (N). Both glycoproteins elicit an antibody response in a person's immune system, i.e. both are antigens. The H protein gets its name because it binds to Red Blood Cells. It is found everywhere on the virus. The N protein is found in clusters on the virus surface; its role is to facilitate penetration into a host cell, once the virus has bound to it.

'Antigenic drift' is the term used for minor antigenic changes. Such genetic mutation is due to selective pressure on the virus from the large population of partially immune people, who have antibodies to the virus as a result of previous infections. This process is continuous and results in local epidemics of influenza. Major antigenic changes (antigenic shift) occur much less frequently. These involve a radical change to either the H or N surface protein. Where the new virus is so different that few or no persons possess immunity to it, a pandemic of life-threatening disease may result.

Three major pandemics have occurred this century - 1918-1919, 1957-58 and 1968-69. The virus that is believed to have caused the terrible pandemic of 1918 has been labeled as the H1N1 virus, it being the first one identified using the techniques of modern microbiology. That of 1957 (the so-called Asian pandemic) involved a change in both the H and N proteins and was classified as H2N2 and that of 1968 (the so-called Hongkong pandemic), which involved yet another change to the H protein, H3N2.

The latter pandemics are relevant to our story because serological studies suggest that the H protein of the virus of the 1957-1958 pandemic was similar to that of the influenza virus that caused the 1889-1890 pandemic, while that of 1968-1969 was similar to the virus of the 1899-1900 pandemic. Somehow viruses from the 19th century managed to survive, and when they returned, there was so little immunity left that they again were able to cause much sickness, worldwide.

Clinical course

The typical course of an influenza infection resembles that of the common cold, i.e. sneezing, coughing, dripping nose, etc., which last for a few days. Additional symptoms in more severe cases include fever, headache, joint and muscle pains. Sydenham in 1679 described influenza that appeared in an epidemic form that year as follows:

> A cough arose ... which seized nearly whole families at once. Some required little medicine, but in others the cough occasioned such violent motion of the lungs, that sometimes a vomiting and vertigo ensued. On the first days of the disorder, the cough was almost dry and the expectoration not considerable, but afterwards the matter in some measure increased ... it was attended with a fever and its usual concomitants ...

The 'typical' influenza is fatal only to the weakest segments of the population, usually confined to the old and very young. The pandemic of 1918-19 differed dramatically from any other pandemic of this or any previous century. Not only was mortality very high, it was a mortality that particularly searched out the strongest members of the age group that hardly is ever affected by influenza, namely those between 20 and 30 years of age.

Death in 1918-19 came mostly from complications of pneumonia. Mortality rates for influenzal pneumonia were more than 60%. The progress of the sickness was so rapid and destructive that first thoughts were that it must be something far more dangerous than the common flu, such as the pneumonic plague. The lungs of those that had died quickly, sometimes less than 48 hours after the first signs of illness, were like no other lungs ever seen in autopsy. The lung tissue lacked any consolidation, having been reduced to a mass of detached pieces floating in a sea of thin, bloody fluid. One hypothesis that explains why the 1918 pandemic was so dramatically different from any other pandemic of influenza is that a mutant form of the bacterium *Haemophilus influenzae* accompanied it.

Typhus

History

The search for typhus in ancient medical texts suggests that it emerged later, perhaps arriving in Europe as late as the 15th century. In the middle of the 17th century Willis noted the presence of what he called a *pestilent fever*, which was contagious and presented with a widespread rash. This was probably typhus.

It was William Cullen (1710-90), professor of theory and practice of medicine in the University of Edinburgh who popularized the name *typhus* in 1769 for fevers that were accompanied by delirium, stupor, or other signs of weakened function of the brain and nerves.[25]

The wars of the 18th century carried typhus far and wide. England was seriously invaded towards the end of that century; it reached the United States early in the 19th century. It should be noted, however, that there is considerable historical evidence suggesting the presence of typhus in South America in earlier, pre-Columbian time.

Countless numbers of devastating epidemics occurred in Europe in the 18th century, mostly in association with famine, the confinement of many people in a small area, and war. In almost every European war typhus took a heavy toll. The French Revolution and the Napoleonic campaigns in Europe, for example, saw more deaths by typhus than by war wounds. England was again heavily infected at the beginning of the 19th century, probably from Ireland, where poor crops and famine had provided ideal conditions for the disease. During the Irish epidemic of 1816 to 1819 an estimated 700,000 cases occurred among the 6 million population. Only towards the middle of the 19th century would the decline in the number of great typhus epidemics in Europe begin.

Etiology

Typhus is caused by one of a group of organisms known as the rickettsiae. Like the viruses, they can grow only in living cells, but they are visible under the microscope. Other rickettsial diseases include Rocky Mountain spotted fever, mite-borne scrub typhus and Q fever. They all are transmitted by insect or related parasites, lice, fleas, ticks or mites, and in some instances through the inhalation of contaminated excreta.

There are two forms of typhus. Its classic form, as it existed in Europe for centuries, is a purely human disease carried from human to human by the louse. The body louse takes up rickettsiae from the blood and transfers the

---

[25] Typhus comes from the Greek word meaning smoke, mist or vapor. Cullen took the name from Boissier de Sauvages who several years earlier had included typhus in his monumental *Nosologia methodica*. Perhaps he was influenced in his choice of words by the Hermetic association between external smokes that overpower the body and internal vapors that overwhelm the brain!

infection to another when it bites again. The louse is fatally infected in the process and lives for only about a week.

The second form of typhus, which is found in the Americas and elsewhere, is transmitted by the bite of an infected flea, which has become infected by biting rickettsiae-carrying rats. There are only slight differences between the rickettsiae that produce the 'rat' and 'louse' infections.

Clinical course

Fracastoro left this account in 1584 of what clearly was typhus:

> for although the heat seems mild for the nature of this fever, however inside the commotion takes possession, & now weakness in the whole body and lassitude, fatigued by nature: decubitus appears on the back, the head becomes heavy, senses are drowsy & the mind for the most part, after the fourth or seventh day, not clear, the eyes redden, many words are spoken, the urine at first pale and very much excreted also enough, soon afterwards red & cloudy, like the urine granatorum: pulse slow & small as we say: the excremanta corrupt, foetid: about the fourth and seventh day red spots on the arms, back & breast, & often they break out red like the bites of fleas, often large, resemble freckles, from which the name was given (lenticulae): thirst either little or none, the tongue grows filthy, somnolence comes to some, wakefulness to others, sometimes in one day by turns: this condition in some until the seventh, others until the fourteenth, others beyond that: the urine in some was suppressed, which was a very bad sign ...

Yellow Fever

History

It is believed that yellow fever originated in West Africa. Its virus cycled between monkeys and mosquitoes usually causing little harm to humans. The first record of a yellow fever epidemic may have been the sickness that killed 200-300 men of Drake's expedition to Cape Verde in 1585. The characteristic yellowish skin, which is due to the liver being infected, gave rise in the 17th century to it being called 'yellow jack'. It spread by means of ships carrying infected mosquitoes or humans or both. It was present throughout the 18th and 19th century world, but limited to where it's vector, the *Aedes aegypti* mosquito, was present, which was primarily in the Americas.

Etiology

Yellow fever is caused by a flavivirus normally transmitted between monkeys by mosquitoes. However, humans are also susceptible to the disease. In the developed urban context, yellow fever is carried by one particular type of mosquito - *Aedes aegypti*. An urban yellow fever epidemic normally involves only humans. Inside African jungles or South American rain forests, mosquitoes that feed on disease-carrying monkeys can infect humans.

Clinical course

Benjamin Rush (see Chapter V), left this description of the 'following marks' that appeared during the course of the 1793 epidemic of yellow fever in Philadelphia:

A yellowness in the eyes, and sallow color upon their skin.
A preternatural quickness in the pulse.
Frequent and copious discharges by the skin of yellow sweats. In some persons, these sweats sometimes had an offensive smell, resembling that of the washings of a gun.
A scanty discharge of high coloured or turbid urine.
A deficiency of appetite, or a greater degree of it than was natural.
Costiveness.
Wakefulness.
Head-ach.
A preternatural dilation of the pupils. This was universal.

Cholera

History

In 1815 the Indonesian volcano Mount Tambora exploded sending 25 cubic miles of volcanic debris into the earth's atmosphere where it disrupted normal patterns of weather. In India, extremely heavy rainfalls followed by disastrous floods and harvest failures marked that year. While the next year was extraordinarily hot and dry in India, New England experienced snow in June and killing frosts that continued through August. In 1817 heavy rainfalls again struck India. This was the year that gave birth to the first cholera pandemic, i.e. worldwide outbreaks.

How these weather changes might have played a critical role in letting cholera escape from what up until then had been its Asiatic home is open to much conjecture. It may have been necessary for the cholera germ to change its form for this escape to have taken place. It seems almost certain that the epidemic form of cholera that swept out of India in 1817 was then what today we would call 'a newly emerging disease', one that was not known to ancient man although there are many ancient references to a disease that carried the name 'cholera'.

The new cholera reached Calcutta in early August 1817; within 3 months nearly all villages and towns of Bengal had been invaded. Although it quickly spread in the immediate areas, cholera did not reach the island of Ceylon until 1819 nor Thailand and Singapore before 1820, and Japan in 1822. Its progress has been linked with military invasions, caravan movements, religious pilgrimages and shipping routes. For example, the cholera invasion of Arabia, which took place early in 1821, has been traced back to the landing of a British expeditionary force sent from India to Oman. In less than three weeks more than 15,000 people died in Basra, the principal port at the head of the Persian Gulf. From here the disease reached northwards passing through Iran and touching the southern shores of the Caspian Sea. It did not progress further presumably due to the severe winter of 1823-24 in Europe.

The second pandemic started in 1826 and was the first to reach the shores of Northern America. Here too it has been possible to trace the spread from area to area and again the only force impeding its progress was the intervening winter, and this only gave a respite for several months each year. The emerging pattern of movement can be likened to the assault of a beach by waves whose height and angle of approach are ever changing. Some parts of the sand are touched immediately, while others are only first reached by retreating waters that have found their way back around and over impeding sand hills. Thus cholera did not reach Marseilles until 1834, arriving there from Spain instead of from other parts of France and two years after it had invaded the distant shores of America.

The next pandemic lasted from 1846 to 1863. It invaded Russia in 1847. There was a lull during the winter, but by December 1848, it had spread to the southern part of the United States. Another quiet spell occurred during that winter and then it spread over the greater part of Europe, involving the whole of France, spreading into North Africa from Italy. In France alone, more than

140,000 people died. On the other side of the ocean, cholera moved by boat from New Orleans to the river Chagres in Panama.

Each successive wave of cholera in the 19th century became more difficult to trace with any degree of accuracy since local outbreaks were composed of a mixture of the new pandemic with still present infections of previous ones. What did clearly emerge, however, was an ever-extending spread of the disease into new areas - Colombia in 1854; Cape Verde islands, Venezuela and Brazil in 1855; and Zanzibar, Bolivia and Peru in 1869. By the end of the century the only places left untouched were the northernmost and southernmost parts of the globe and remote areas not reached by any commercial, religious or military contacts.

Etiology

Cholera is caused by the bacterium *Vibrio cholerae*, which can be present in untreated water contaminated with human excrement. The vibrios are swallowed in contaminated water or food and multiply enormously in the intestine. Only some strains of *V. cholerae* are able to produce cholera. Each pandemic is caused by a new epidemic strain.

Clinical course

A clinical case of cholera begins when the bacteria colonise the human intestine. The irritant substances produced by the vibrios alter the physiology of the lining of the intestine, allowing fluids to leak into the intestine. The immediate result is a catastrophic watery diarrhea. Acute spasmodic vomiting and painful cramps are generally present. Dehydration is great and often accompanied by cyanosis. Death may occur with no warning and within hours of the first appearance of symptoms.

During the second pandemic, the following description of its course was published in an English journal to help the public recognize the disease that was new to them:

> *... giddiness, sick stomach, slow or small pulse, cramp at the top of fingers and toes ... Vomiting or purging of a liquid like rice-water ... the face becomes sharp and shrunken, the eyes sink and look wild, the lips, face, neck, hands and feet, and the whole surface of the body a leaden, blue, purple, black ... The skin is deadly cold and often damp, the tongue always moist, often white and loaded, but flabby and chilled like a piece of dead flesh. The respiration is often quick but irregular ... urine is totally stopped.*

Typhoid

History

The clinical characteristics of typhoid resemble those of other diseases so there is little certainty that any of the ancient texts actually describe it. Some scholars have 'found' typhoid in passages in the bible as well as in Hippocratic texts. But the earliest sure description of typhoid dates from the mid-17th century when Thomas Willis differentiated typhoid clinically from other fevers, giving it the name *putrid fever*.[26] The evidence for Willis' knowledge of typhoid has recently been strengthened by the discovery of Christopher Wren's drawings of a typhoid ulcer, signed by him and Wren.

Many clinicians continued to confuse typhoid with typhus so that even a picture of its recent history is difficult to construct. Nevertheless, by the end of the 19th century it became evident that typhoid was one of the chief causes of fever in the cities throughout the world, appeared as a special problem in times of war, and caused sporadic outbreaks in rural populations. The American Civil War, where typhus was strikingly unimportant, saw an estimated 75,000 cases of typhoid.

Etiology

Typhoid is caused by the bacillus *Salmonella typhi*. It enters the body by ingestion. Multiplication of the invading organism occurs in the small intestine during an incubation period of 10-14 days. Humans are the only reservoirs for the disease and most infections are transmitted by the fecal contamination of food or water by those sick from typhoid or by chronic carriers, who otherwise appear healthy.

Clinical course

The vivid (but partial) description left by Willis from a publication dated 1684 is of interest in that it mixes a description of the fever with his interpretation of how the body's humors are involved:

---

[26] Willis also described the lesions of the ileum produced by typhoid, likening them to the lesions of smallpox. Paradoxically, this later gave rise to the suggestion that the two diseases were the same, and that all smallpox vaccination did was to suppress skin manifestations while increasing the likelihood of internal damage. Those who opposed smallpox vaccination added this belief to argue against it.

When therefore any one is taken with a putrid fever, the first assault is for the most part accompanied with a shivering or horror: for when the blood begins to grow hot, there is a flux made, and a swelling up of the crude juice, freshly gathered together in the vessels, even as in the fit of an intermitting fever, heat, and sometimes sweat follow, upon the shivering, by which, the matter of that crude juice is inkindled, and dispersed: afterwards, a certain remission of the heat follows, but yet from the fire still glowing in the blood, a lassitude and perturbation with thirst and waking, continually infest: a pain arises in the head, or loins, partly from the ebullition of the blood and partly from the motion of the nervous juice being hindred; also a nauseousness, or a vomiting offends the stomach, because the bile flowing out of the choleduct vessels, is poured into it, and a convulsion form vapours, and from the sharp juice brought thorow the arteries, is excited in the stomach.

Epidemic Puerperal Fever

History

Puerperal fever was first described by Hippocrates. But it does not seem that its epidemic form existed before the mid-seventeenth century, when "*an unknown affection,*" that occurred at Leipzig in 1652 attacked puerperal women and "*was so deadly that but one in ten escaped.*" The next epidemic is recorded to have taken place during the winter of 1746, when there was an epidemic at the Hôtel-Dieu in Paris. The first English epidemic was in 1760. Virulent epidemics continued until 1936 when maternal mortality fell with the introduction of the sulfonamides.

Etiology

Puerperal fever may be caused by different organisms, the most common of which is the *ß-haemolytic streptococcus*. This highly infectious agent attacks the uterus of postpartum women. In the absence of sterile procedures, most infectious bacteria enter from the outside during a medical intervention. Occasionally, the genitalia's own bacteria may be harmful.

Clinical Course

Peripartum infections are often manifested by fever and bacteremia. Although these infections typically produce only mild symptoms, occasionally patients have severe and sometimes rapidly fatal sepsis.

Part III - 18th and 19th CENTURY HISTORY

V

18th Century - A Kind of Status Quo Reigns

In Europe, epidemics of infectious diseases were much less serious and much less widespread in this century than in the previous one. Malaria, influenza, and scarlet fever were common, as were diphtheria and smallpox. Typhus was present under various names and epidemics of yellow fever occurred but limited to various parts of the New World. Plague and syphilis were much less malignant but serious epidemics of the former still did occur on occasion.

The 18th century differed from previous ones in other important ways. Religious differences still existed but major wars over those differences had died out as religious divisions in Europe solidified. A period of 'enlightenment' ensued, one that was dominated by the positive belief that scientific knowledge could be used to improve man. In France, the medical professions even went so far as promoting the radical idea that modifying his social and cultural environment could perfect man's temperament.

Despite the dramatic social, cultural and economic changes and great advances in science that took place during this century, little progress was made concerning the understanding of what caused epidemics. It would even be difficult to point to any development upon which the real progress of the 19th century rested, other than basic progress in chemistry and physiology, including the development of improved tools. For all intents and purposes, an ill-defined 'status quo' reigned, centered on the essential idea of 'tainted air' or 'charged atmosphere'.

In this chapter we explore the 'status quo' through an examination of a combination of specific epidemics and theories concerning the spread of diseases. The reader will find in the latter many remnants of Hippocrates as well as the newer ideas introduced during the prior centuries by Fracastoro, van Helmont, Fludd and others.

Plague in Marseilles: 1720-22

The most likely cause of the plague, as far as I'm concerned, is the poisonous emanations from underground vitriolic and arsenic mines, which pushed by a central fire rise into the atmosphere where they are received by those

> *living there who in turn communicate the disease to their neighbors and from one country to another. (Brother Victorin, Marseilles, 1721)*

During the Black Death of 1347-1350 Marseilles lost four-fifths of its population by 1348. Severe outbreaks again occurred in the 17th century. In 1628 plague carried off half the population of Lyons, and one million died in northern Italy in the next years. It spread through Germany and the Netherlands, struck Eastern Europe in 1654, and reached its terrible climax in London's Great Plague of 1665, when possibly 75,000 died.

The epidemics of plague in the 18th century were still frequent but on the whole less virulent than in previous centuries. Still, bubonic plague killed more than 300,000 in Prussia in 1709. As reflected in the introductory quote, thinking concerning the origin of plague had not advanced from the time of the Black Death. All one could hope to prevent its arrival was an effective system of quarantine. Attempts to create such a system followed the 1719 peace treaty between the Ottoman and Habsburg Empires. The latter erected a huge *cordon sanitaire*; 4000 men controlled a 1200-mile frontier, supported by several thousand more when the intelligence service noted plague in the East. Travelers along with their animals and goods were then quarantined and disinfected.

Marseilles was one such City to have a *cordon sanitaire* in place when the ship *le Grand Saint Antoine* approached the French coast in May 1720. This was its return voyage from Syria, where it had picked up a shipment of very valuable cotton. It departed from Syria on 5 February and stopped in Tripoli on 3 April, where several Turkish passengers boarded, one of who died two days later. It then made a rest stop in Cyprus from 7 to 18 April. Between 27 April and 17 May there were four more deaths on board including that of the ship's surgeon. On arrival at Livourne on 17 May three further deaths occurred. The sanitary authorities at Livourne labeled the deaths *"suspicious,"* so the ship's captain did not go directly to Marseilles but instead made an illegal stop near Toulon where he contacted the ship owners to inform them of the situation. They in turn contacted the owners of the cargo, one of who was the first alderman of Marseilles.

Le Grand Saint Antoine finally arrived at Marseilles on 25 May where it was put into quarantine. Since the cotton was to be sold at a major fair in the coming weeks, pressure was placed on the sanitary authorities and, owing to the influence of the first alderman, quarantine was lifted from the ships cargo on 3 June, well in advance of the normal forty days called for. In spite of the fact that one more death occurred on the ship 12 June, passengers were allowed to disembark on the 14th.

The first suspicious death in Marseilles itself occurred on 21 June. Nearly each new day saw another death, several of which were individuals who had bought cloth that had been stolen by the sailors to sell as contraband. On 9 July two doctors announced the presence of plague to the town's aldermen. Immediately the traditional anti-plague measures were started - bodies were buried at night in quicklime, houses where any deaths had occurred were walled-in and their occupants taken to the infirmaries, and a strict surveillance was established to isolate the town's hospitals. By 15 July Marseilles was obliged to tell other ports of the outbreak, but at the same time they sought the advice of a surgeon. He declared that the disease was only an 'ordinary' fever.

The heavy rains of 21 and 22 July were a prelude to fourteen deaths on the 23rd of that month. Still the surgeon, Bouzon, indicated that it was not plague; nevertheless, the town authorities took further steps to stop its spread. The town's beggars were housed together, while 3000 foreign beggars were forced to leave. On 31 July, the parliament of the region placed a ban on Marseilles but, by then, an estimated 10,000 people of Marseilles' 100,000 population had already fled the town, carrying plague with them to other parts of France.

A *cordon sanitaire* was established on 4 August around Marseilles. 89 posts were established on the roads leaving the town, manned by 281 farmers, 332 soldiers and 31 officers. The death penalty was levied for any communication between Marseilles and the rest of the Provence. In October a nearly 100km long plague wall (Mur de la Peste) was erected across the countryside, north of Marseilles. The wall was built of dry stone, 2 m high and 70 cm thick, with guard posts set back from the wall.[27] Meanwhile the situation in Marseilles rapidly collapsed becoming more nightmarish with each passing day. By 9 August the cemeteries were full and the hospitals were no longer accepting any new cases. Bodies started appearing on the streets, and the means to bury them were totally overwhelmed.

---

[27] Parts of this wall still remain and can be seen in the Plateau de Vaucluse.

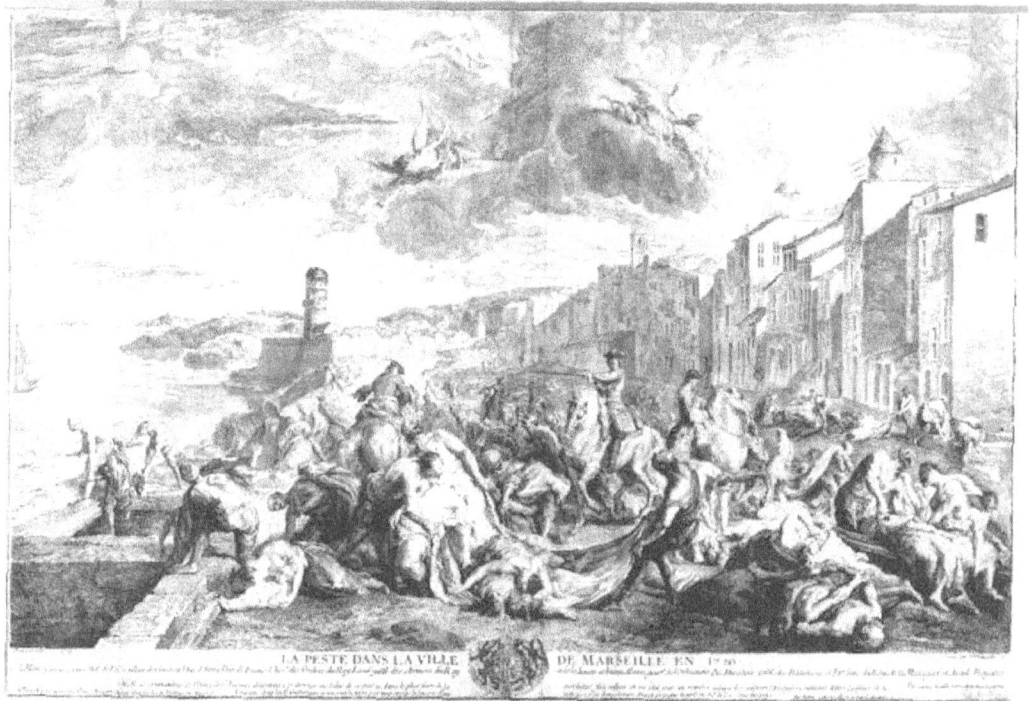

LA PESTE DANS LA VILLE   DE MARSEILLE EN 1720

On 15 August an official medical commission from Montpellier established after 24 hours of investigation that it was indeed plague. By this time the mortality rate had reached 400 per day. To avoid adding to the growing panic, the official announcement was only that of a *"contagious malign fever."* However, nothing could be hidden from the populace. The number of deaths per day grew steadily along with the pile of bodies left to rot on the streets. By the end of August there were more than 1000 deaths occurring each day and in the old town there were 7 to 8 thousand cadavers that were being devoured by wild dogs. Nearly everyone who could flee had already done so. The list of officials still in place could be counted on two hands.

Efforts to clean the streets of dead bodies proved nearly impossible to organize and fatal to almost all that tried. On 16 September 40 volunteer soldiers leading 100 prisoners and wearing head masks soaked in vinegar managed to clean one particularly dreadful town square. Of that group, only five of the volunteer soldiers did not contract plague and die. By this time, nearly 30,000 had died in Marseilles alone.

It was only in late October that some normalcy returned. The death rate had dropped to less than 100 per day. Looters were arrested; foreign doctors were no longer needed; the bourgeoisie emerged from their homes; people started to look for jobs again. There was a flurry of marriages, especially among those who had lost their spouse. However, when one party was recovering from any sickness, they were obliged to pass a medical examination before the marriage could take place.

Plague faded as rapidly as it had come. Although it would return again in May 1722 the greater damage had already been done. Nearly 60% of the population of Marseilles had been stricken with plague, and of these some 80% had died, resulting in nearly 50,000 deaths, or half of the town's population.

England Awaits the Plague

The shrieks of women and children at the windows and doors of their houses, where their dearest relations were perhaps dying, or just dead, were so frequent to be heard as we passed the streets, that it was enough to pierce the stoutest heart in the world to hear them. Tears and lamentations were seen almost in every house, especially in the first part of the visitation; for towards the latter end men's hearts were hardened, and death was so always before their eyes, that they did not so much concern themselves for the loss of their friends, expecting that themselves should be summoned the next hour. (Defoe)

Not surprisingly, the outbreak in Marseilles caused grave alarm in England. The plague of 1665 was part of London's living memory. For those who were too young to remember, Daniel Defoe's *A Journal of the Plague Year*, published in 1722, from which the above quote was taken, provided an all-too-vivid account of that calamity. Defoe had been reporting on the threat of plague from 1719 when it first appeared in Hungary. A steady stream of his articles described plague in Marseilles and other parts of southern France.

The hero of Defoe's *Journal* is a saddle-maker who by want and necessity observes and reports on the progress of plague as it moves from one end of London to the other. His initials are H.F., which are thought to stand for Henry Foe, an uncle of Defoe who may very well have been in London in 1665. Through a detailed accounting of the published weekly bills we learn of the number of burials by parish and disease. The drama of whole families being kept imprisoned in their houses when any member is found sick is particularly striking.

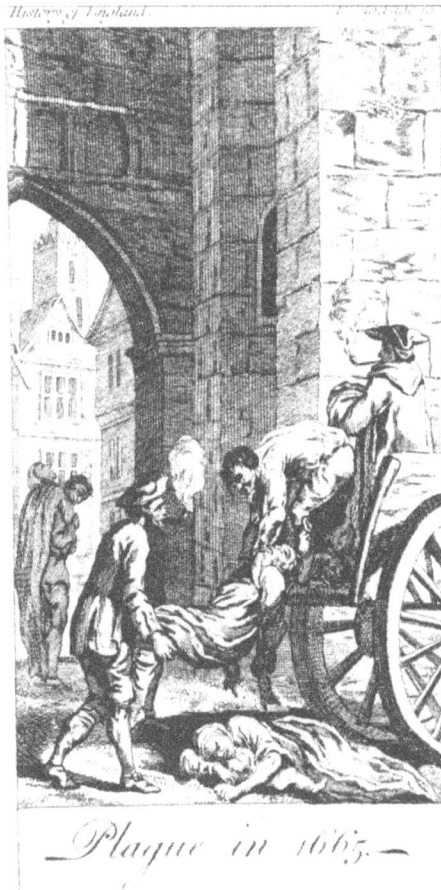

Plague in 1665.

We learn of a blazing star or comet that had appeared for several months before the onset of the epedimic , as well as one that passed one year later just before London's great fire.[28] The two comets _"passed directly over the city, and that so very near the houses that it was plain they imported something peculiar to the city alone."_ Other signs included _"the conjunctions of planets in a malignant manner and with mischievous influence."_ H.F. saw both comets and had to confess that he looked upon them _"as the forerunners and warnings of God's judgments."_ At the same time he was aware that astronomers assigned natural causes for such events, knowing how _"their motions and even their revolutions are calculated."_ That the disease might have resulted from an _"immediate stroke from Heaven,"_ however, he looks upon with _"contempt as the effect of manifest ignorance and enthusiasm."_

Although lacking any medical training, H.F. volunteers his thoughts concerning how plague spread:

---

[28] Boyle, for example, believed that God was the first cause of things and is ever present. Comets and other _"irregularities in the cosmos"_ are examples of events he attributed to an active God. Thus it was logical to attempt to interpret these events as messages from God. Even after Newton had demonstrated that the motion of comets followed the laws of gravity there still remained room for imagining the origin of such events as being under the immediate control of God.

...the calamity was spread by infection; that is to say, by some certain streams or fumes, which the physicians call effluvia, by the breath, or by the sweat, or by the stench of the sores of the sick persons, or some other way, perhaps, beyond even the reach of the physicians themselves, which effluvia affected the sound who came within certain distances of the sick, immediately penetrating the vital parts of the said sound persons, putting their blood into an immediate ferment, and agitating their spirits to that degree which it was found they were agitated; and so those newly infected persons communicated it in the same manner to others.

I look upon with contempt ... the opinions of others, who talk of infection being carried on by the air only, by carrying with it vast numbers of insects and invisible creatures, who enter into the body with the breath, or even at the pores with air, and there generate or emit most acute poisons, or poisonous ovae or eggs, which mingle themselves with the blood, and so infect the body.[29]

one man who may have really received the infection and knows it not, but goes abroad and about as a sound person, may give the plague to a thousand people, and they to greater numbers in proportion, and neither the person giving the infection or the persons receiving it know anything of it, and perhaps not feel the effects of it for several days after.

H.F. contemplates this latter possibility further by posing the questions - *"how long it may be supposed men might have the seeds of the contagion in them before it discovered itself in this fatal manner, and how long they might go about seemingly whole, and yet be contagious to all those that came near them."*

H.F.'s medical friend, Dr Heath, suggests that those infected *"might be known by the smell of their breath; but then, as he said, who durst smell to that breath for his information?"* A safer possibility was that infected breath might be distinguished *"by the party's breathing upon a piece of glass, where, the breath condensing, there might living creatures be seen by a microscope, of strange, monstrous, and frightful shapes, such as dragons, snakes, serpents, and devils, horrible to behold."* No microscope was available with which to make this experiment. After some further suggestions are explored, H.F. concludes - *"But from the whole, I found that the nature of this contagion was such that it was*

---

[29] This may have been directed to Richard Bradley, an English botanist, who in his 1721 publication *The Plague of Marseilles* linked the plague with air being filled with *"vast varieties of the smaller kinds of insects."*

impossible to discover it at all, or to prevent its spreading from one to another by any human skill."

Defoe was a firm believer in angels and the devil, and accepted as true some accounts of apparitions.[30] He placed Satan not in Hell but *"sitting in great state, in open campaign, with all his legions about him, in the height of the atmosphere ..."* So it would have come as little surprise if he had chosen to account for plague along supernatural lines that many of his compatriots had followed during the previous century. But his particular puritanical beliefs greatly reduced his options. While he believed, for example, that angels possessed foreknowledge, he also believed that God denied them the use of that knowledge to warn communities of impending disasters. If God chose to act he does so largely by *"notices, omens, dreams, hints, forebodings, impulses, etc ... a kind of communication with the invisible world, and a converse between the spirits embodied and those unembodied."* From these, the *"prudent man (can) foresee the evil, and hide himself."* And although angels were able to control the forces of nature, scientific measurement of such phenomena as the weather and the passage of comets suggested that they were no longer inclined to demonstrate their force as they had in biblical times.

On the other hand, Defoe totally disapproved of the use of charms and talismans. This *"kind of astrological magic"* was the work of the devil. He condemned it *"as being a plain robbing of Providence of its known glory, in directing and disposing both causes and events in all things relating to the government of mankind ..."*

Defoe's plague texts touched on many questions that preoccupied the medical community. Richard Mead (1673-1754), for example, who was asked by the English government in 1719 to report on the matter, referred to Defoe's work *"as an authority."* This is not too surprising given the fact that Defoe had based virtually his whole account on historic fact.

Mead was one of London's leading medical practitioners and a friend of Alexander Pope, Edmond Halley and Newton.[31] Although not familiar with

---

[30] He published in 1726 his *Political History of the Devil* and its sequel *A System of Magick, or a History of the Black Art.*

[31] In an earlier work, *On the Influence of the Sun and Moon upon Human Bodies and the Diseases Thereby Produced*, Mead, on the basis of Newtonian mechanics, argued that the sun and moon produced changes in atmospheric pressure which determined the amount of nervous fluid in the human body and, thus, receptivity to disease.

the disease himself, Mead had access to previous reports to the Government and available literature on English and European epidemics. His initial report was a small pamphlet of 7000 words (later editions were considerably longer). The first third was devoted to *Nature of Contagion* and the last two-thirds to *Methods to Prevent Contagion*.

There was no place in Mead's accounting of plague for the 'wrath of God'. He drew upon Hippocrates' dictum that no sickness was more divine than any other. He could not believe that God was directly responsible for epidemics, since there could be no way *"whereby his vengeance might be distinguished from common events"* resulting in the *"innocent (being) equal sharers with such calamities with the guilty."*

Mead identified three primary causes - the air, diseased persons and goods transported from infected places (fomites). He was very aware that there were some who thought that the disease was so infectious as to leave no role for the air, while others ignorant of the potential for infection ascribe plague wholly to air's *"malignant quality."* His aim was *"to make a proper balance between these two, and to set just limits to the effects of each."*

Plague will never be great enough *"to load the air with infectious effluvia"* to the degree that it *"could be conveyed by the winds into a neighbouring town or village."* But those individuals *"very near to the sick Person"* could be infected by the *"active particles"* thrown off by the body, particularly *"those of the mouth and skin, from which the secretions are naturally the most constant and large."* The *"conveying of mischief to a great distance from the diseased body"* calls for both the body to be emitting much more active and powerful infectious matter and the air to be corrupted enough *"to give these contagious atoms their full force."* Otherwise, *"it were not easy to conceive how the Plague, when once it had seized any place, should ever cease."*

Having conceived the *"matter of contagion"* to be an *"active substance, perhaps in the nature of a salt."* Mead had no difficulty in conceiving how such a substance *"may be lodged and preserved in soft, porous bodies, which are kept pressed close together."*

In short:

> The Plague is a real poison, which being bred in the southern parts of the world, is carried by commerce into other countries, particularly into Turkey, where it maintains itself by a kind of circulation from persons to goods ... When the constitution of the air happens to favor infection, it rages there with great violence: that at time more especially diseased

persons give it to one another, and from them contagious matter is lodged in goods of a loose and soft texture, which being packed up and carried into other countries, let out when opened the imprisoned seeds of contagion, and produce the disease whenever the air is disposed to give them force.

Based on these conclusions Mead had little choice but to advise a system of quarantine, which in its specifics resembled those to be found on the continent. A new Quarantine Act, replacing that of 1710, was rushed through parliament in the winter of 1720-1.[32] Stiffer penalties were introduced along with new provisions permitting the establishment of a military *cordon sanitaire* around any infected town. Magistrates could compel the moving of infected individuals into pesthouses. The death penalty could be invoked for any disobedience.

Mead's text did not please everyone. At the political level, there was strong repugnance to the strong-handed way in which the government could interfere in everyday life. While such power might be acceptable to the people of France, they were intolerable to people under a 'free government' in England. The government was forced to reconsider. A new Quarantine Act was enacted in February 1722. The quarantine of ships remained but the government could no longer quarantine towns or force the sick to be moved against their will. Nor were death penalties prescribed for any disobedience.

Mead's text also attracted considerable opposition from his medical colleagues, particularly those who opposed quarantine. One direct medical attack came from a young physician, George Pye, in his *A Discourse of the Plague wherein Dr Mead's Notions are Consider'd and Refuted*, one of the few tracts that attacked Mead directly. Pye denied plague could be passed from person to person, arguing instead that plague was fully miasmatic in nature, an affliction that arose from local circumstances, depending more on the disposition of the air than on *"effluvia from the bodies of men."* Other critics agreed - plague originated locally; an extensive and hard quarantine was not required.

John Arbuthnot (1667-1735), a physician and friend of Mead, observed that plague occurred more or less at the same time in places widely apart from each other and concluded that only a *"universal cause"* could account for such

---

[32] This act replaced the first quarantine act, which had been passed in November 1710. Some believe that the earlier act was first suggested by the writer Jonathan Swift who had heard that plague was present at Newcastle.

a thing. He proposed *"the hypothesis of extraordinary effluvia."* Citing the plague of 1346, he noted how it had begun in the Kingdom of Cathay as a *"vapour most horridly foetid, that breaking out of the earth, like a kind of subterraneal fire, consumed and destroyed above 200 leagues of that country ... and infected the air."* The infected air then went on rapidly to Greece and the rest of Europe.

Many physicians took the time to report on their own views concerning plague. Not all were driven simply by economic considerations that dominated the anti-quarantine faction. For example, Joseph Browne wrote *A Practical Treatise on the Plague* where, while lauding the work of Mead, he used the occasion to resurrect ideas that earlier writers had proposed, many of which he felt Mead should have paid more attention to. In fact, Browne had expected a more *"elaborate treatise"* from *"so learned a pen as yours,"* especially when *"all the eyes of the people of Great Britain look steadfastly on you, as one from whom they may expect deliverance."* Perhaps it was this sort of criticism that led Mead to greatly expand his later treatises while not, however, changing his basic ideas concerning causation.

Browne wanted two other causes to be added, namely *"diet, and diseases that are the causes of other diseases."* Diet, because ...

> it affords matter to the juices ... (and) the more a man eats, the less he perspires; the less he perspires, the more danger there is of a plethora. Again, all things that subject to fermentation are bad, and all things which relax the tone, and incline it to flatulencies, diarrhea's and all putrid diseases which arise from too great plenty of serum.

He illustrated *"diseases that are the causes of other diseases,"* including the *"propagation of the disease itself towards another,"* as follows:

> too large an hamorrhage from the nostrils, disposes the parts to vertigo or apoplexy. Colliquative sweats relax the tone of the parts, hinder digestion, and promote the hectick. Obstructions of the bilious ducts, produce the black and yellow jaundice, inflamations of the stomach, vomiting, and spasmodick contractions of the heart. A cachexia in acute fevers, will beget a malignity, a malignity in putrid ones the plague; for when the status of the blood and serum is corrupted, there happens a defection or want of strength and spirits, loss of sense, coldness of the extreme parts, and burning within, a weak, flow and unequal pulse.

Browne reminded Mead of the work of Kircher and others which implicated insects and *"animated or living putrefaction,"* including the possibility that the *"air might be demonstrated to be verminous by the microscope."* More importantly,

111

he noted that such contagious particles *"could not fix their malignity upon the stomach, or convey it immediately to the blood ... were there not some latent seeds of the same malignant nature inherent in the body before."*

Browne was not sure were such latent seeds come from. This he left for Mead's *"more accurate decision."* He did, however, have some thoughts on the subject himself:

> *But that diseases have in them some such influence or magnetick-like attraction, seems to me plain from some hereditary ones that are propagated from father to son, and which lie a long time unseen, unfelt, and closely couch'd within the bed of nature; that is, are lock'd up in the viscidity of the blood, Lympha Saliva, or other juices of the body, and at last break out according to the force of the active principle.*

Browne even evoked the possibility of a latent seed being aroused by *"the very thoughts of an approaching mischief:"*

> *when a timorous person hears a relation of a malignant small pox or plague, and the terrible symptoms attending them, he immediately forms to himself a perfect idea of that disease, which rouzes in his blood a malignant ferment or contagious seed, which seizes on the vital spirit, and there the conflict is begun and carried on, till one or the other conquers.*

More generally:

> *The contagious atoms that are diffus'd through the air, and are wafted up and down with every blast in pestilential seasons, and infected places, tho' slightly entering into the body unfelt, unseen, cannot of themselves make the plague, unless the constitution of the body happens to favour the infection; which, with humble deference to your learned judgment and opinion, is quite the opposite to your assertion.*

* * * * *

Fortunately for England plague did not arrive in the 1720s and, as noted earlier, with few exceptions, it was not to be seen in Europe again.

Later in the century, the American epidemiologist, lexicographer, educator and patriot Noah Webster (1758-1843) published his *History of Epidemic and Pestilential Diseases* in which he devoted some space to plague. His analyses of past plague texts led him to be severely critical of Mead's report, indicating that it was the *"weakest and least valuable performance on the subject now extant."*

Webster noted that there was an interval of six weeks between the great London plague of 1665 and the half-dozen cases that had occurred in 1664. From this he argued against the imported nature of the disease as follows:

> *The suspension of the disease, during six weeks, is evidence that infection had no agency in spreading the disease. It is a fact known and acknowledged, that infection cannot be preserved, for a tenth part of that time in the open air. Air dissolves the poison of any disease, in a very short time. Infection can only be preserved in confinement, as in close vessels or packages of goods. The walls of an infected house will be cleansed by the action of air, in a very few days, so as to be perfectly harmless. During the six weeks suspension of the plague in London, where was the infection concealed to preserve it from air and frost?*

Furthermore, his belief that no case of plague had occurred following the great fire in London in 1666 supported his view that the 'cause' of plague had been removed:

> *The old city of London was **contrived**, one would think, to breed plagues. The streets were winding and narrow - the houses high and the upper stories jutted over the streets so that they almost met from opposite sides and covered the street below, - add to this, the want of good water. How could such a place escape the pestilence? By fire.*

Referring to the outbreak in Marseilles, Webster argued forcefully against the view that the infection had been introduced on an incoming ship. *"How in the name of reason,"* he asked, *"could men or goods be infected, when the disease did not exist in the place?"* Furthermore, since Webster believed that there had been a period of six weeks between the last death on the ship and the recognition of the disease in Marseilles, he concluded that it was *"clearly impossible that there could have been any propagation of the distemper by infection."* He went on to predict that *"it will probably be proved, that the plague generally if not always originates in the country where it exists as an epidemic."*

The writings of Defoe, Mead, Pye, Arbuthnot, Browne, and Webster offer a full range of disease causation possibilities. None were ruled out. The authors differed essentially on which factor or factors to give greater priority. Pye and Webster highlighted the local origin of plague, while Mead and Arbuthnot paid greater attention to how plague propagates from one place to another. For Arbuthnot, the mode of propagation was through the movement of the air, while for Mead, it was mostly *"contagious matter lodged in goods."* For all, the local air must *"be disposed"* to the contagion for it to start and continue. But

Browne placed greatest emphasis on the body being ready to receive the infection, either by poor diet, conditioning diseases or the presence, possibly through inheritance, of plague seed. It would also seem that all believed that once the local air no longer supports any further spread, plague must die out.

Hardly any attention was given to the possibility of a "*healthy carrier*" of disease. The exception was Defoe's H.F. who contemplated the possibility of men going about "*seemingly whole, and yet contagious to all those that came near them.*" Then current notions of disease did not support such a belief since disease was essentially defined in terms of abnormal signs and symptoms, i.e. one could not be whole and diseased at the same time.

We will come back later to both Arbuthnot's and Webster's beliefs concerning the origin of epidemic diseases when we review the outbreaks of influenza that occurred towards the century's end. Webster is also important as an influence on Benjamin Rush, a key figure at the end of the 18th century.

Tuberculosis - The Ignored Ideas of Benjamin Marten

The doctrine of the contagiousness of the disease (tuberculosis) has ... its advocates, but general belief is in its non-communicability. (1881 Medical Textbook)

In 1720, Benjamin Marten, an obscure English practitioner published a remarkable book entitled *A New Theory of Consumptions: More Especially of a Phthisis or Consumption of the Lungs.* Marten specified *phthisis* in the title to distinguish his subject from other wasting diseases, e.g. diabetes, cancer, and abscesses of the lungs. For Marten, tuberculosis was not due, as others claimed, to "*a serious disposition of the juices ... a salt acrimony ... a strange ferment ... a malignant humor*" but rather to "*some certain species of Animalculae or wonderfully minute living creatures that, by their peculiar shape or disagreeable parts are inimicable to our nature; but, however, capable of subsisting in our juices and vessels.*"

Marten was aware of the invisible world that microscopes had opened up. Antony Van Leeuwenhoek (1632-1723) had introduced the term *Animalculae*. Leeuwenhoek communicated his microscopic discoveries to the Royal Society of London from 1673 to several months before his death. He described what in time would come to be realized to have been protozoa and bacteria in the human mouth and intestine, but he never himself conjectured his 'little animals' as the cause of disease.

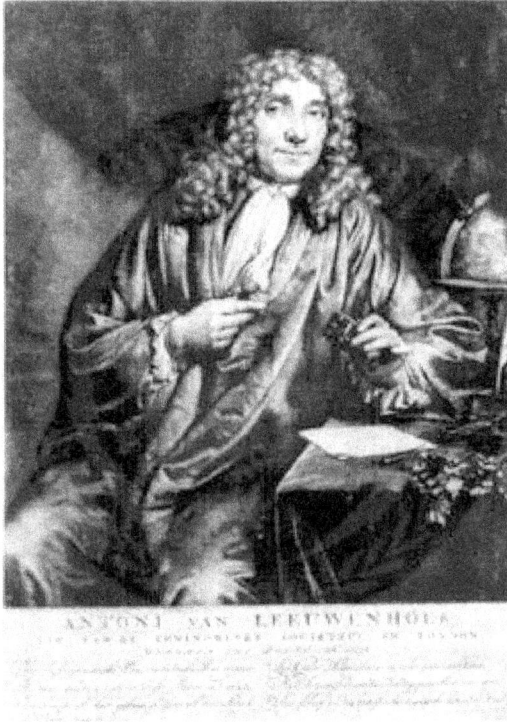

ANTONI VAN LEEUWENHOEK

Not only did Marten think it possible that tuberculosis was caused by *"minute animals or their seed,"* he also suggested that it could be passed on either from parents to their offspring *"hereditarily"* or *"communicated directly from distempered persons to sound ones who are very conversant with them."* He advised against lying in the same bed with a consumptive patient or conversing with them *"so nearly as to draw in part of the breath he emits from the lungs."* The similarity between Marten's ideas and those of Browne are evident. But whereas Browne included the seeds of plague as but one of many possible means whereby plague might be transmitted, Marten focussed on only that possibility for tuberculosis.

Marten's work attracted little interest but it did reach Boston, where it had a receptive reader in Cotton Mather, as discussed below. Mather knew of Marten's animaculae just as well as the general public probably did. Joseph Addison (1672-1719) had written about the microscopic world in an essay in the *Spectator*, a popular paper issued between 1711 and 1713. He pointed out that there is not a single *"humour in the body of man … in which our glasses do not discover myriads of living creatures."* But rather than imagine that these creatures might cause disease, as Mather did, Addison extolled *"the exuberant and overflowing goodness of the supreme being,"* and even suggested that this finding enhanced the likely existence of angels or other beings above man, *"since there is an infinitely greater space and room for different degrees of perfection between the supreme being and man, than between man and the most despicable insect."*

That the goodness of God could be witnessed in the plenitude of creatures that inhabited the universe was an idea that had deep historical roots. Augustine, for one, saw in the variety of the things that had been created out of nothing, "*the supreme art of God.*" Sometimes referred to as The Great Chain of Being, the basic argument was that God had created a universe in which a hierarchy of all possible creatures resided, including heavenly objects. Earlier we referred to Fludd's belief that the sun occupied the midpoint of this chain where others placed man. However conceived, most chains, like that of Addison, left far more space between man and God than below man, or as Locke put it:

> *We have reason to be persuaded that there are far more species of creatures above us, than there are beneath; we being in degrees of perfection much more remote from the infinite Being of God, than we are from the lowest state of being, and that which approaches nearest to nothing.*

This belief possibly contributed to less attention being given the 'small'.[33] It seems that it was easier to contemplate the angelic and demonic creatures in the heavens than it was to speculate on what could not be seen even after Leeuwenhoek's observations of *Animalculae*. Also contributing to Marten's failure to gain attention with his ideas was the fact that his work had been published when London was being threatened by plague. However, his medical colleagues were aware of his 'new theory'. They simply chose to ignore it. When his book was rediscovered in 1911, only four copies of it could be found and almost nothing concerning its author.

Martin, himself, recognized that his 'new theory' challenged the humoral tradition of disease; only when the latter was abandoned did he feel that his theory would gain acceptance. Instead, as we will explore at the beginning of Chapter VI, humoral theories gave way to other physiological theories, and the role of external seeds, germs, and animaculae, as such, remained on the sidelines for another century.

* * * * *

Had Marten been born in either Italy or Spain, his book probably would have suffered a much better fate. In both of those countries tuberculosis was firmly

---

[33] On the other hand, Sydenham imagined that - "*Nature performs her operations on the body by parts so minute and insensible that I think noebody will ever hope or pretend even by the assistance of glasses or any other invention to come to a sight of them and to tell us what organicall texture or what kinde of ferment ... separate any part of the juices in any of the viscera.*" At the same time, however, he regarded the use of the microscope as immoral and outside God's purpose.

thought to be contagious, so much so that anatomists avoided performing autopsies on patients dead of phthisis to avoid contacting the disease. Fracastoro, as already noted, had written about its contagiousness in 1546.

In 1699, the Republic of Lucca promulgated the first anti-tuberculosis legislation which gave directives to protect citizens from being *"harmed or imperiled by objects remaining after death of a person suffering from phthisis,"* and ordered physicians to notify the government of all cases *"treated for the suspected malady."* Physicians of Naples issued a statement that left little doubt concerning their beliefs:

> *Pulmonary consumption is of such a malignant nature in our country that even after the death of the sick person the seed of his malady remains hidden and unseen in many houses, with serious danger to those who move into them thoughtlessly; and indeed some of this seed is so penetrating that it can be communicated even without immediate contact with the infected person or thing.*

Some believe that the law in Spain against the emigration of consumptive individuals is responsible for the fact that the Indians colonized by the Spaniards remained free of tuberculosis longer than those that had been colonized by either the English or the French.

English and French physicians, along with those from other North European countries, seemed to base their anti-contagion theory for tuberculosis on the hereditary nature of the disease. Only certain families seemed to suffer the most, and within families, very similar histories could be found, for example, brothers and sisters becoming consumptive at almost the same age.

American physicians, almost all trained in Northern European schools, followed suit, as can be seen from the introductory quote which is taken from the fifth edition of the textbook *The Principles and Practice of Medicine* written by August Flint and William H. Welch. There, the causes of tuberculosis are *"hereditary disposition, unfavourable climate, sedentary indoor life, defective ventilation, deficiency of light and depressing emotions."* It will be noted that this book was published only one year before Robert Koch's discovery of the bacillus of tuberculosis!

Cotton Mather Battles Smallpox

'Tis the Destroyer, or the Devil, that scatters Plagues about the World. Pestilential and Contagious Diseases, 'tis the Devil who does oftentimes invade us with them. 'Tis no uneasy thing for the Devil to impregnate the Air about us, with such Malignant Salts as meeting with the Salt, of our Microcosm, shall immediately cast us in to the Fermentation and Putrefaction, which will utterly dissolve all the Vital Tyes within us...And when the Devil has raised those Arsenical Fumes, which become Venemous Quivers full of Terrible Arrows, how easily can he shoot the deleterious Miasms into those Juices and or Bowels of Mens Bodies, which will soon Enflame them with a Moral Fire! (Mather, 1692)

It begins now to be vehemently suspected that the Small-Pox may be more of an animalculated Business than we have been generally aware of. The Millions of ... which the microscopes discover in the Pustules, have confirmed the suspicion ... (Mather, 1724)

In Cotton Mather (1663-1728) we find a religious zealot who actively participated in the 1692 Salem witch trials and a natural philosopher who fought against religious and medical opposition in order to introduce vaccination against smallpox in 1721 when an epidemic broke out in Boston. In one man, thus, we find the deadly intolerance of the Reformation and inquisitive openness of the Enlightenment.

Mather entered Harvard at the age of 12 and received his MA degree at 18 from the hands of his father, Increase Mather (1639-1723), who was then president of Harvard College. Unlike his father, who travelled to and lived for a while in England, Cotton lived all his life in Boston. There, he read extensively and corresponded regularly with the Royal Society of London. He was awarded an honorary degree from Aberdeen in 1710 and his publication *Curiosa Americana* won him membership in the Royal Society in 1713.

The Mather library became one of the largest private libraries in the Colonies. Cotton, who had given some thought to becoming a physician before he became a Congregational minister, was responsible for most of the medical works acquired. These included, among many others, the familiar names of Hippocrates, Paracelsus, van Helmont, Boyle, Kircher, Sydenham, Willis, Mead and Martin.

From his extensive readings Mather acquired a broad view of medical theories then prevalent on the Continent, as reflected in the opening quote concerning the workings of the Devil! He wrote extensively on medical matters, but most of this material was scattered widely in various pamphlets. Only towards the end of his life did he pull this material together into the unpublished book, *The Angel of Bethesda*. Although Oliver Wendell Holmes found Mather's medicine *"absurd,"* this book provides an extraordinary summary of the major competing theories of disease causation.

Of the multitudinous ways that disease could invade the body, Mather became in time particularly attracted to those that were evoked by the microscopic world of Leeuwenhoek. Drawing on the works of Marten, Mather described this world as follows:

> *Every Part of Matter is peopled. Every green Leaf swarms with Inhabitants. The Surfaces of Animals are covered with other Animals... As there are infinite Numbers of these … so there may be inconceivable Myriads yett smaller than these, which no Glasses have yett reach'd unto. The Animals that are much more than thousands of times less than the finest Grain of Sand, have their Motions... The Eggs of these Insects (and why not the living Insects too!) may insinuate themselves by the Air, and with our Aliments, yea, thro' the Pores of our Skin; and soon gett into the Juices of our Bodies.*

Smallpox was a major killer in the Colonies. Mather had lived through the severe outbreak of 1678 when the only means of defence were isolation of individuals and materials, and calling upon God for forgiveness of whatever sins that had brought this plague upon the community. He rejected the view that smallpox was an ancient distemper that is passed from generation to generation through *"the Maternal Blood"*, lying *"dormient and buried, until it be fired by Contagion..."* Instead, as noted in the second opening quote, he believed smallpox to carried by some form of animaculae.

Mather held that the severe form of smallpox entered the lungs through respiration from where it was carried directly by the blood to the surrounding organs, particularly the heart, where it did immediate harm.

When introduced by inoculation, however, the *"Miasms of Small-Pox"* had a longer route to take before it could reach the heart, by which time it would be greatly attenuated and thus less likely be the cause of severe damage:

> *The Enemy, tis true, getts in so far as to make some Spoil; yea, so much as to satisfy him, and leave no Prey in the Body of the Patient for him afterwards to seize upon. But the vital Powers are kept so clear from his Assaults, that they can manage the Combats bravely and, tho' not without a Surrender of those Humours in the Blood which the Invader makes a*

Seizure on, they oblige him to march out the same Way he came in, and are sure of never being troubled with him any more.

Mather first learned of the practice of inoculating people with smallpox from an African slave who had witnessed it in African villages. Several articles he received from Europe provided much more detailed descriptions of how that practice was carried out. Thus, he was fully prepared to promote its use when smallpox broke out in Boston in early 1721.

Mather proposed to the physicians that they undertake inoculation, but only Zabdiel Boylston (1680-1766) accepted. The others *"treated the Proposal with an Incivility and an Inhumanity not well to be accounted for."* It seems he had less opposition from his clerical colleagues.

Boylston first tried it out on his only son, a boy of thirteen, and two Negro slaves, a man and a boy. They suffered no ill effects nor did they get smallpox when later exposed to patients suffering that disease. By September he had inoculated 35 persons with no deaths. All told, he inoculated 247 people in Boston; another 39 were inoculated by other physicians. Six of the inoculated group died. The epidemic caused 5729 cases of smallpox among the near 10,000 population of Boston, of which 844 died. Many of the survivors were disfigured with scars and broken in health.

Boylston and Mather were confronted with critics even while the epidemic was still raging. Boylston was attacked in the street and both he and Cotton Mather had bombs thrown into their homes. Even though the death rate of those inoculated was far less than those who contracted the full disease, Boylston was accused by some of murder. Medical opposition, led by William Douglass, the only Boston physician with an MD degree, feared that, uncontrolled, inoculation threatened to spread disease. As its effectiveness became more evident and controls over its use were installed, the opposition faded and inoculation became generally accepted.

As a devote Calvinist, Mather believed that the cause of all illness was punishment for sin. That he now believed that some form of animaculae caused smallpox raised a serious theological problem. He solved that problem by holding that God must have created these germs for the very purpose of punishing sinners:

What unknown Armies has the Holy One, wherewith to chastise ... the rebellious Children of Men? ... Billions or Trillions of Invisible Velites! Of sinful Men they say, Our Father, shall we smite them? On His order, they do it immediately; they do it effectively.

Mather's solution to this theological question would have been severely questioned on the Continent where a parallel but related question was being hotly debated among theologians, namely whether human parasitic worms, e.g. intestinal worms, 'spontaneously' generated in the human body or entered it by unknown means.

Antonio Vallisnieri (1661-1730), an Italian physician, who believed that intestinal worms were created when man was created and had inhabited the human body ever since, realised that this raised the question when did God create these worms. It was not *"reasonable to suppose that God would have placed the first worm in his (Adam's) body, forasmuch as Man in this state of innocence was to be free of all kinds of diseases."* But if created after the fall of Man, then an even greater difficulty presented itself, since *"God hath taught us, that before Man was made, all other animals were created."* He resolved this problem by proposing that before Man's fall these same worms did good works, e.g. *"by gently licking the parts (of Adam) and by healing them..."* Only after the Fall did the worms alter their role. But others pointed out that, before the Fall, Adam was in a state of perfection that would require no such beneficial assistance![34]

With the exception of specific points of opposition, for example, as existed in Calvinist Scotland where the clergy resisted inoculation on the ground that it interfered with God's Providence, inoculation with human virus gained ground in the colonies and in Europe only to be replaced towards the end of the century by inoculation with cow-pox virus, which was introduced by Edward Jenner (1749-1823), an English physician, in 1798.

---

[34] The history of spontaneous generation as it applied to worms is somewhat different than that of microorganisms. Worms, it was believed, derived from living organic matter. Found inside humans, it was virtually impossible to demonstrate that they had not generated 'spontaneously' since there was no way to deprive the human body of all possible sources with which they may have entered the body. Belief in their spontaneous origin existed well into the 19th century up until the time when pathological anatomy began to have a better understanding of the human infections associated with hydatid and other tapeworm cysts.

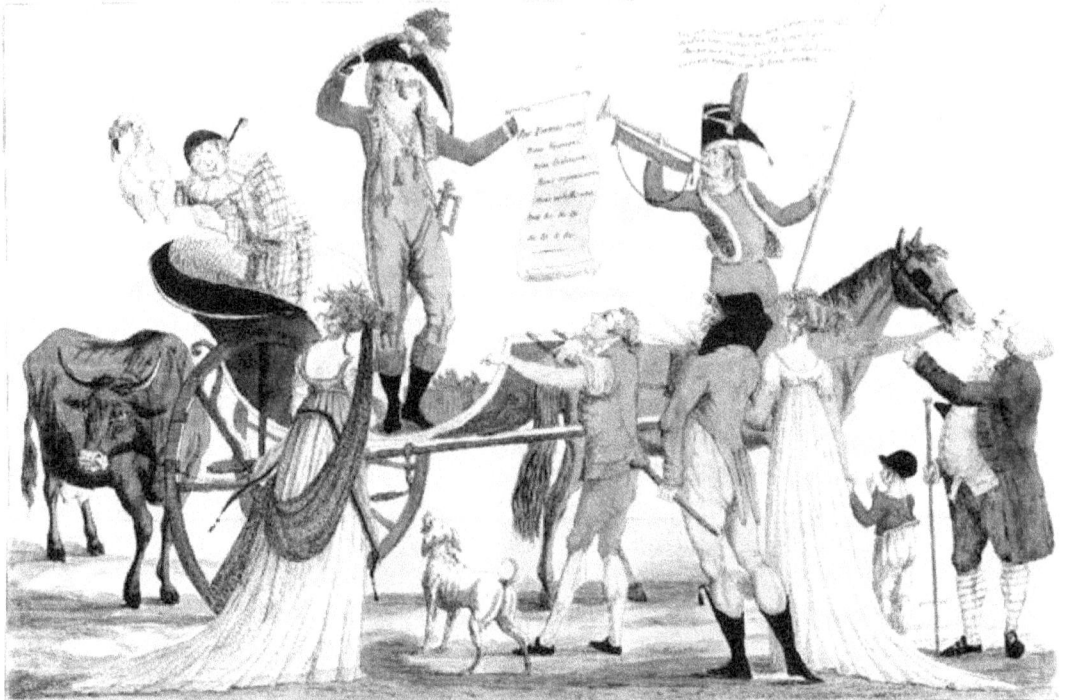

LA VACCINE EN VOYAGE.

Diphtheria in the American Colonies: 1736-40

We are led to look beyond natural Causes to the Hand of God, to whom we are chiefly concern'd to apply our selves for the removal of this awful Calamity. (Fitch)

The Reverend James Fitch, pastor of the North Church in Portsmouth, New Hampshire, spoke these words in 1736 during the second year of the 'throat distemper' outbreak. Spring had come late the previous year; the weather was unusually wet and cold.

On 20 May 1735, the town of Kingston witnessed its first fatality, Parker Morgan, who died after a brief illness. A week later, 3 children died within three days in a house on the other side of town. All 3 seemed to have suffered the same illness. In the month that followed, 13 other children died, more deaths than usually occurred in a whole year. 19 more succumbed in July. By the end of December, the death toll reached 102. The epidemic would continue for three more years; by the end of 1738, the sickness had visited nearly every family in the community, and more than a third of all the children in the town had died. Of the first 40 who were taken ill, not a single one recovered. Many died within twelve hours, some of them *"while sitting up at play with their playthings in their hands."*

The outbreak was a complex one, involving **both** scarlet fever and what would come to be known as diphtheria in due course (see Chapter VI). All parts of New England were touched between 1735 and 1740. In some of the towns nearly half of the children died. Diphtheria seemed to have had two, possibly three, points of origin, one in New Hampshire, the other in New Jersey, and the third, assuming it did not originate in New Jersey, in Connecticut. The course of scarlet fever is not known with any certainty. It seemed to be widely present, sometimes concurrently with that of diphtheria, sometimes alone.

New England was used to many different diseases, some of which particularly attacked children. There had been outbreaks of whooping cough, measles, smallpox, dysentery and influenza. But none had lasted this long nor had been this mortal, and none before had reached across nearly all of the inhabited regions of the area. Previously there had been some mention of scarlet fever and a few descriptions of cases that might have been diphtheria, but there had clearly never been this kind of outbreak before. No call was made for applying existing stringent laws to prevent the spread of smallpox and other contagious diseases, since this new disease did not spread like the others. It attacked here and there, jumping towns, missing some families while decimating others. It baffled local physicians, appearing as it did in different areas with no apparent pattern.

Special fast and prayer days were proclaimed and the public was called upon to humbly reflect upon the *"especial sins which God is angry with."* Lamentations and poems were written to record the agony of suffering and the helplessness of the physicians, whose art *"can find no part, nor cure for this distemper."* Fitch, when he found from his studies that the disease vented its fury chiefly upon the children, attributed it to *"the woeful Effects of Original Sin."*

Puritans believed that they were involved in a binding contract or 'covenant' with God. Failure on the part of any individual to obey his laws could result in the whole community suffering the wrath of God. Children were not exempt. On the contrary, as Cotton Mather wrote in 1689, children *"go astray as soon as they are born.*" They need to live in order to redeem themselves. That so many died young was both an indication of 'original sin' and a general failure on the part of the community to adhere to the terms of their covenant with God.

Boston was aware of the outbreaks that had occurred in nearby New Hampshire and awaited this new disease with some apprehension. The smallpox epidemic of 1721-2 was still fresh in the minds of many. The intervening fifteen years since that outbreak had been one of rising prosperity and good health; the town selectmen naturally wished to avoid another siege of sickness. In early October 1735 they called upon the medical community to advise how best to protect the public from the ravages of "*the throat distemper.*" The group of physicians that met would later organize the first medical society in America. After considerable discussion and some consultation with doctors in nearby towns that had seen several cases, they concluded that "*the said Distemper was communicated by means of a bad Air and not by Contagion.*"

By November of that same year, it became clear that the throat distemper had actually invaded Boston but at a rate much slower than had been the case in the smaller towns of New Hampshire. First cases seemed to have occurred the previous August. Deaths mounted slowly during the winter, but almost miraculously, most of the Boston children quickly recovered from their illnesses. Mortality was much less than what had been experienced earlier. By April the selectmen were proclaiming through the newspapers "*that scarce any Distemper, even the most favorable which has at any time prevailed, so generally, has produced fewer Deaths.*" The epidemic reached its peak in March of 1736; by its conclusion later that year, it was supposed that one-fourth of all the people of Boston had contracted the disease, and that out of 4000 cases, 114 had died.

The medical community of Boston concluded that their superior abilities were responsible for the lower rate of mortality observed! They were aware that in their cases a rash occurred while no such rash was present in those of the country towns. They concluded that some "*morbifick matter*" in the blood caused the distemper and that it was only necessary to prescribe some efficacious remedies that would allow the poisons to reach the skin surface, evaporate through the pores, and thereby produce a rash. Successful treatment resulted in the rash; their New Hampshire colleagues had failed to bring out that rash in their patients, thus explaining their high fatality rate.

Boston doctors appear to have been treating scarlet fever while New Hampshire was under assault by diphtheria. The confounding of these two diseases was not surprising. They would be taken to be the same disease for at least another century. Diphtheria is a disease that may appear in many different ways. In some it takes the form of a simple head cold, while in others it is an affliction of the skin. In its most fatal form, individuals may suffocate within a few hours of first symptoms. That it might also cause a scarlet rash to appear is not so out of the question. It would only be in the early part of the 19th century, as discussed in Chapter VI, that diphtheria would be separated from scarlet fever and the other diseases with which it was confused.

Malaria in the Roman Campagna

A horrid thing called mal'aria, that comes to Rome every summer and kills one. (Horace Walpole, 1740)

During the 15th, 16th and 17th centuries Rome was infected with all sorts of epidemics and stricken with famine after famine. Malaria, which was always present, began to take on a more fatal form towards the end of the 16th century and proved far more serious than plague and other epidemics during the 17th and 18th centuries. Agriculture in the surrounding areas of Rome was completely ruined by the epidemics of fever. Some villages that had had populations of more than 1000 inhabitants in the 14th century had dwindled to just over 100.

In general, 'the fever' was associated with water, swamps and air. Summer and autumn rains were feared as an increased number of cases always followed them. Giovanni Maria Lancisi (1654-1720), physician to Pope Innocent XI, published his famous book concerning malaria in 1717, *On Harmful Emanations from Swamps, and on their Remedies.* He prescribed the following rules to prevent "*the pernicious effects of exhalations rising from morasses in hot climates:*"

1. Care should be taken that the bed chambers do not face the south.
2. That the door and windows be not left open.
3. That the rooms be aired with resinous or scented wood, or with sulphur.
4. He advises to eat and drink sparingly; but of wholesome food.
5. To make the sauces acid with lemon and pomegranate juice, or vinegar.
6. Not to go abroad with an empty stomach.

7. To use cooling liquors.
8. To avoid the night air and keep at home in the morning till sun rises.
9. To forbear all violent exercise.
10. Not to swallow the saliva or spittle.
11. To carry a sponge moistened with spirits of wine and a theriacal vinegar, and often to smell it.
12. To keep the mind calm and free from anxious solicitudes and violent passions.

Lancisi accused Gregory XIII, who was Pope briefly in the 12th century, of having made a *"great error"* when he cut down a large wood lying to the south of Rome, a wood which in the past had kept *"off a great part of the noxious vapours."* The danger of the south winds were so well known that travelers to the Campagna were advised not to pass a night there *"before the North wind has purified the air."* Intriguingly, Lancisi also gave some thought to the possibility that mosquitoes might be the cause of malaria. He also advanced the theory that malaria might be caused by a parasite, suggesting that the blood of patients suffering from fever be examined microscopically. Writing of the mosquitoes, he suggested that *"they inoculated their own bad humors into our blood."*

Lancisi produced sketch maps of marshes and wind directions and was responsible for early attempts at draining the Pontine Marshes. One can see in his list of advice specific points that applied to both disease transmission possibilities, i.e., that of contaminated air as well as disease- (bad humors) carrying mosquitos. In comparison to his attention to epidemiology, climate and terrain, little space is allotted in Lancisi's book to therapeutics. He allowed for two methods, bleeding and the Peruvian bark.

The Peruvian bark had entered Europe during the first half of the previous century and was only just beginning to be recognized as a powerful anti-malarial treatment at the time of Lancisi's book. A more important book, strictly dedicated to the usage of the bark had been published in 1712, namely *Therapeutice specialis* by Francesco Torti.

As already noted briefly at the end of Chapter III, physicians totally dedicated to the Galenic school of treatment resisted the introduction of the bark. It will be remembered that Hippocratic teachings indicated that acute illnesses, especially those that are accompanied by fever, are resolved by coction - cooking or digestion - of the causative humors. In favorable cases, a crisis would be reached followed by the discharge or evacuation of the residues of the coction process. Peruvian bark violated this most basic tenet of Hippocratic medicine, in that there was neither a crisis nor much evidence of any residue being discharged or evacuated.

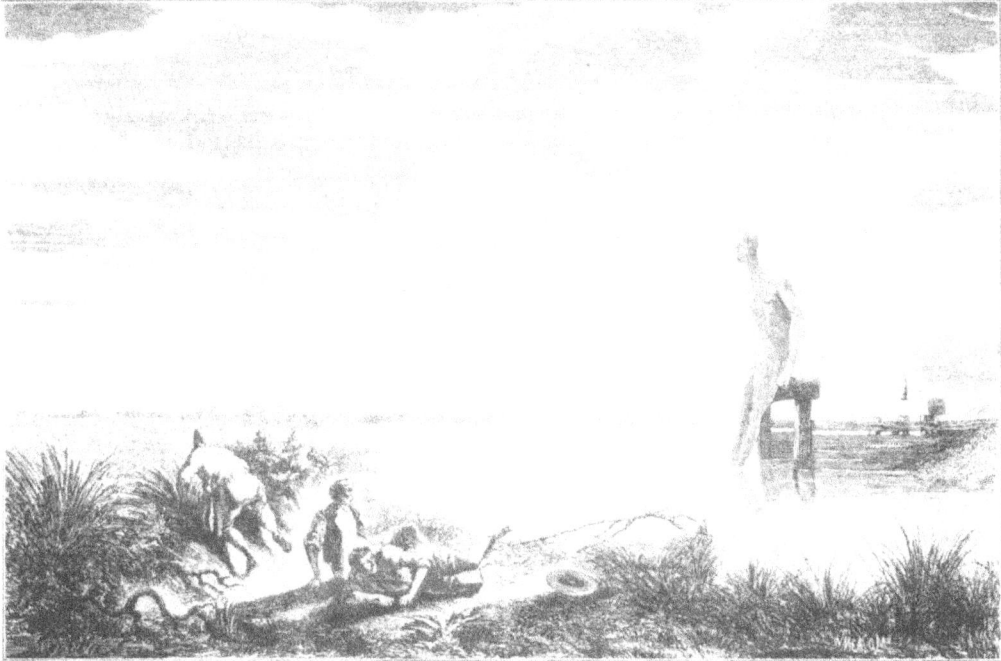

Maurice Dudevant   The Ghost of the Swamp

Already in 1656, one medical writer had observed:

and so we see that China Chinae (the name by which the bark was best known in Italy at that time), a unique prodigy in medicine, overthrows and tramples to the ground not only the quartan fevers, based on cold humor, but also tertian fevers, which are based on hot, dry, and bilious humor, and we see also that the China is inherently hot and dry.

In 1663, one physician, still clinging to the traditions of Hippocrates, was forced to conclude *"the bark must be judged to operate by hidden qualities rather than by manifest qualities, as happens also in syphilis ... for guaiac works by hidden qualities."*

A second cause of opposition lay in the fact that the tertians seen by Hippocratic physicians were not dangerous and that the crisis seen in that disease would appear around the seventh bout with fever. As noted in Chapter IV, the tertians of Hippocrates were limited *to P. vivax* infections. The malignant tertian, i.e. *P. falciparum* infections, were not yet present in Europe. Waiting for the 7th cycle of fever in a case of falciparum malaria would have been a sure way to invite death.

The use of the bark gained general acceptance as it proved to be both safe and effective. Malaria epidemics, however, after a slight slowing down in the middle of the century, returned to their earlier high levels. The agricultural and commercial Congress in 1794 offered a prize for the best method of overcoming malaria. The most important prophylactic measure remained the lighting of fires at nightfall to surround dwellings, as ordered by Pius VI, Pope from 1775 to 1799.

Typhus in England

Nervous, putrid, bilious, petechial or miliary, they are all of the malignant family; and in this great town (London) they are almost the only fevers that have for many years prevailed, and do so still, to the great destruction of mankind. (Armstrong, 1773)

Typhus fever is a disease of overcrowding and poverty. (Encyclopedia Brittanica 1876)

Before it was pathologically disinguished in the early 19th century, it had been seen as a multitude of diseases. In the 16th century it was identified in terms of the spots it produced (e.g. *lenticulae*, spotted fever, flea-bite fever[35]), while later it was in terms of the conditions where it struck (e.g. gaol fever, famine fever, hospital fever, ship fever, camp fever, Irish ague). It was present in all corners of England throughout the 18th century but appearing in epidemic form only on occasion and mostly confined to overcrowded and poor situations.

---

[35] One might have imagined that this association with fleas would have sped up the identification of the louse in the transmission of typhus. In fact, early in the 17th century Tobias Coberus hazarded the idea of a relation between typhus and lice but his suggestion was not taken seriously.

As implied in the words of Armstrong, an army physician, fevers were more often than not named according to their physiological consequences. Distinguishing typhus from other forms was not possible with any degree of certainty. However, some mortality figures did separate out 'spotted fever' from the more general category of 'fever'. As to its cause, aside from its link with crowding and poverty, no consistent picture emerged. During a 1741 outbreak among weaving towns, one medical writer ascribed the outbreak to bad bread. But a Birmingham surgeon took exception and fell back instead on the words of Sydenham - "*a contagious quality in the air, arising from some secret and hidden alterations in the bowels of the earth ... or to some malign influence in the heavenly bodies.*"

One observer even suggested that the air could be made 'pestiferous' by the perspiration of people! He calculated that 2904 individuals during a 34 day period would perspire enough to cover an acre of ground with 1 inch deep of "*perspired matter ... which, rarefi'd into air, would make over that acre an atmosphere of the steams of their bodies near 71 foot high.*" This would turn pestiferous unless it was carried away by the wind.

The close association of typhus with crowded and dirty conditions prompted some in the 18th century to instigate sanitary measures well before any of the fever diseases had been correctly distinguished. James Lind (1716-1794), perhaps best known for having introduced citrus fruit to combat scurvy in the British navy, came to see typhus (ship fever) as a disease carried not only on the bodies of men, but upon clothes, on all kinds of materials and even upon furniture and wooden beams (i.e. fomites).

Lind had been greatly impressed by a devastating outbreak of what resembled ship fever in 1746 among the Mimack Indian nation in Nova Scotia. The outbreak resulted from a party of Indians distributing blankets and old clothes that they found by accident and that had been discarded by the French following an outbreak on their ships. Lind pushed for fumigation and ordered thorough scouring and cleansing, and removal of bedding and all clothing to the decks to be sunned and aired. He recommended that physicians and nurses change their clothing when leaving the hospital. For newly recruited sailors, he ordered for their clothes to be baked. He fought for an increase of soap allowances among the troops.

Lind linked jail conditions with outbreaks on ships. He observed in his 1757 publication on the *health of seamen*:

The sources of infection to our armies and fleets are undoubtedly the jails: we can often trace the importers of it directly from them. It often proves fatal in impressing men on the hasty equipment of a fleet. The first English fleet sent last war to America lost by it alone two thousand men.

Lind showed to John Howard (1726-1790) a number of sailors in one hospital ward ill of the gaol fever that had been brought on board their ship by a man who had been discharged from a prison in London. Howard knew from first hand experience both the horrors of prisons and the sub-human conditions that could prevail on ships, having himself been captured in 1754 by a French privateer while travelling on a British merchant ship and then transferred to a French dungeon where he was treated with great severity.

When Howard became High Sheriff of Bedford in 1773 he began his career as a prison reformer. He visited prisons not only in his area of jurisdiction but throughout England and many other countries on the continent including Russia. On each visit he recorded his observations. Almost all prisons brought evidence of jail fever. A typical entry read:

Between first visit in 1775 and next on 5 Feb., 1779, the surgeon and two or three prisoners have died of the gaol-fever. In 1775 a prisoner discharged from the gaol went home to Axminster, and infected his family, of whom two died, and many others in that town afterwards.

Through his efforts acts were passed that required the walls and ceilings of prisons to be scraped and whitewashed at least once a year, rooms to be regularly cleaned and ventilated, infirmaries to be provided for the sick and proper care to be taken to get them medical advice. Howard, himself, was to die of typhus contracted during a visit to Russian military hospitals.

Another dramatic outbreak of typhus linked with jails was the so-called Black Assizes that occurred in 1750 in Old Bailey. This was a court session of intense local interest so the courthouse was extremely crowded. Within at most a week or ten days following the session many people were "*seized with a fever of the malignant kind, and few who were seized recovered.*" This is taken from a report of one of the justices of the King's Bench, who then went on to observe:

The putrid effluvia which the prisoners bring with them in their clothes etc., especially where too many are brought into a crowded court together, may have fatal effects on people who are accustomed to breathe better air; though, the poor wretches, who are in some measure habituated to the fumes of a prison, may not always be sensible of any great inconvenience from them.

Following this and other similar outbreaks the physician Sir John Pringle (1707-82) and the physiologist Stephen Hales (1677-1761) were asked to advise on how to purify the air of Newgate prison to prevent jail fever. Newgate was London's main criminal gaol, and came to symbolize all that was wrong with 18th century English prisons. Pringle and Hales recommended the reinstallation of ventilators that had been used earlier in the 1740s. Several such devices were installed but results were less than convincing. It was rumored that when the windmill ventilation device was installed in 1752 two men fell dead when the first blasts from the exhaust pipe struck them! Prisoners claimed that their "*healthiness*" had improved, but cases of jail fever still kept occurring.

The measures advocated by Lind, Howard, Pringle and Hales were part of a general move towards 'cleanliness' in which they played a critical part. These measures must have saved lives but being largely confined to military and prison establishments the common man, living in crowded, filthy and under-ventilated conditions, still suffered greatly. One small step that was taken, however, but only in 1803, that improved ventilation in all buildings, not only prisons and hospitals, was the alteration of the Window-Tax that the government had passed in 1746.

A tax on the number of windows in an establishment was first passed in 1696. It was written in such a way as to apply to the whole establishment and thus fall primarily upon the owner to pay. In 1746 the new law levied the tax on individual windows, thus making it easier for the landlords to charge the tax directly to tenants. Howard noted the effect of the tax both in the prisons and in homes:

> *The gaolers have to pay it; this tempts them to stop the windows and stifle their prisoners ... This is also the case in many work-houses and farm-houses, where the poor and the labourers are lodged in rooms that have no light nor fresh air; which may be a cause of our peasants not having the healthy ruddy complexions one used to see so common twenty or thirty years ago. The difference has often struck me in my various journeys.*

Lind, who had been one of the earliest proponents of the use of ventilators, later came to view them as having little effect on the spread of disease.

New-Gate

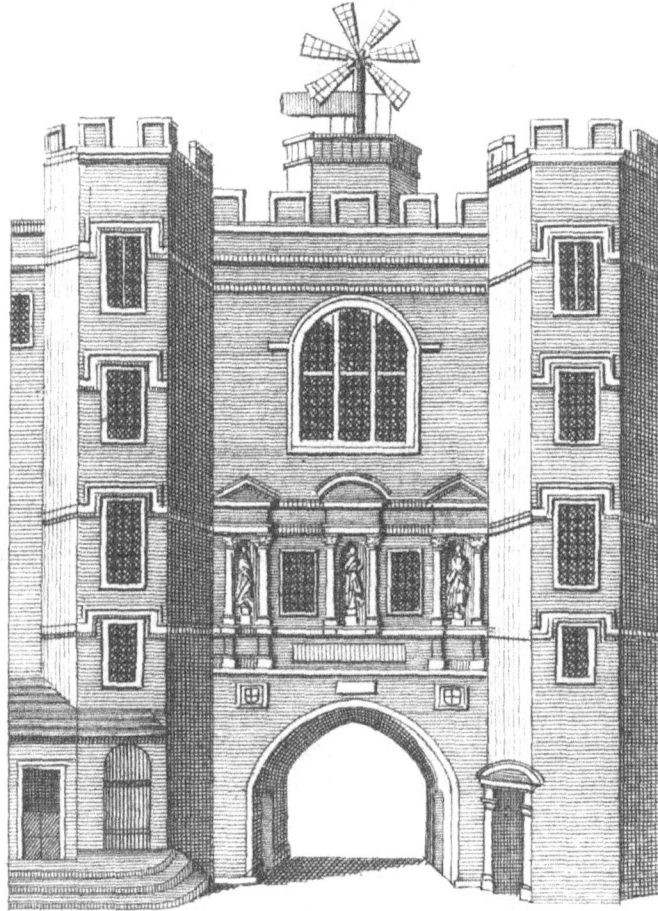

Influenza - The Views of Arbuthnot and Webster

Nothing accounts more clearly for epidemical Diseases seizing Human Creatures inhabiting the same Tract of Earth, who have nothing in common that affects them, except Air. (Arbuthnot, 1733)

All the great plagues that have afflicted mankind, have been accompanied with violent agitations of the [meteorological and geological] elements. (Webster, 1799)

Arbuthnot had occasion to witness the influenza pandemic of the 1732-33 winter, while Webster was present during that of 1789-90. While Arbuthnot's analysis was confined to the 1732-33 epidemic, Webster studied all previous outbreaks, especially that of 1781-82. In London, Arbuthnot noted that for about three weeks in January 1733, the Bill of Mortality was higher than any time since the 1665 plague. During the 1781-82 pandemic two-thirds of the population of Rome and three-quarters of that of Munich were estimated to have fallen sick. Although this pandemic is ranked as one of the most widespread and dramatic outbreaks of the disease, mortality was low, restricted mostly to the old and those sick with chronic respiratory illness. All pandemics followed the familiar pattern of starting somewhere in the East and reaching the West over water and land trade routes.

By the time of the 1781 pandemic, most European specialists agreed that influenza's origin lay beyond Russia, somewhere in India or China and possibly Japan. Webster, however, argued that the origin of it and the earlier 1732-33 pandemic was American, since in both instances there had already been an earlier outbreak on the East Coast of America! He conjectured that the disease had traveled west across the American continent, the Pacific and onto China from whence it continued across Russia to Europe.

Arbuthnot linked the outbreak of influenza in Western Europe with local climatic conditions. He noted that the *"previous constitution of the air"* throughout most of Europe during the fall of 1731 *"was ... a great drought."* There were frequent fogs but they did not bring any form of precipitation - *"rain, snow, or any other fruits of the air."* *"Southerly winds and stinking fogs"* dominated for some time, leading, as surgeons noted, to *"a great disposition in wounds to mortify."* Spring was unusually warm and accompanied by *"great quantities of sulphureous vapours, producing great storms of wind from the South-west, and some lightning without thunder."*

How did these conditions produce disease? For Arbuthnot, it was the *"ill constitution of the air."* Already in the fall, it had proved *"noxious to animal bodies ... a madness among dogs; the horses were seiz'd with the catarrh before mankind."*[36] The effect of the drought was to open up the earth's surface from

---

[36] Early literature often noted concurrent flu epidemics among humans and animals, with outbreaks among animals sometime preceding that of humans. Horses were named most of the time but dogs and cats were also occasionally mentioned. Later other domestic and wild animals were added, in particular pigs and ducks, which today are recognised as major carriers of flu and even sources of new forms of the virus.

which *"new effluvia hurtful to human bodies"* could emerge. These were the *"thick and stinking fogs which succeeded the rain."* These effluvia, not being of *"any particular or mineral nature were watery exhalations,"* ones that are *"hurtful to the glands of the windpipe and the lungs, and productive of catarrhs."*

Arbuthnot is classified in the Encyclopaedia Britannica as a *"physician and wit."* Early in his career, he supported himself by teaching mathematics. His medical career included his having been the royal physician in ordinary to Queen Anne. He is probably best known to the public for his fictitious history of John Bull published in 1727 with a preface signed by both Pope and Swift.

Following Sydenham and Boyle, Arbuthnot developed a general theory of epidemics which he incorporated in his *An Essay Concerning the Effects of Air on Human Bodies* published in 1733. He proposed that physicians should identify those qualities of the atmosphere with *"a power of producing diseases."* In general, he held that effluvia emanating from the earth might combine with atmospheric or meteorological properties and qualities to cause epidemics. He allowed for emanations from diseased persons of from other contaminated sources to create an epidemic-supporting atmosphere.

Webster, like Arbuthnot, was gifted in many different ways. Initially he trained to practice law, but legal prospects not being favorable at the time, he took up a career as a schoolmaster. While teaching, he published *A Grammatical Institute of the English Language* in three parts, a spelling book, a grammar and a reader. Over 15 million copies of the spelling book were sold during the author's lifetime, providing an income that allowed him to pursue other scholastic ventures including the study of epidemiology and the preparation of his well-known dictionary.

His interest in epidemiology was first aroused during the influenza epidemic of 1789 and 1790. The 1793 outbreak of yellow fever in Philadelphia (discussed below) furthered his *"curiosity with double zeal."* After publishing a collection of papers concerning this disease, he turned his attention to other epidemics both in America and throughout the world. His *History of Epidemic and Pestilential Diseases* was published in December 1799.[37] It had neither popular nor medical success, but as discussed below, it did have an important influence on the thinking of Benjamin Rush, a leading medical authority of that era.

---

[37] Osler called this work *"the most important medical work written in this country by a layman."*

One of Webster's essential arguments was that epidemics were the product of a *"pestilential state of the air,"* which often could extend over the whole earth. The violence and extent of these epidemics depended on the number and violence of certain phenomena - *"earthquakes, eruptions of volcanoes, meteors, tempests, inundations."* He calculated that in the 17th and 18th centuries there were 67 records of comets and 85 of volcanic eruptions, with which he associated 179 periods of special prevalence of disease.

Influenza illustrated perfectly an example of a disease determined by the epidemic constitution of the air. It could not be contagious since so many people are stricken *"in a day without any intercourse with each other."* It was the disease *"most closely connected with pestilence and the least dependent on local causes."* Its astonishingly rapid spread over land and sea was most readily explained by some unknown *"insensible qualities of the atmosphere,"* which he believed to be an *"alteration in the chymical properties of the atmosphere,"* electrically determined in association with changes in the inner fires of the earth.

It easily followed, according to Webster's thesis, that the severe pandemic of influenza experienced by Europe in 1781 had its origin in a much milder form of the disease that had been present in America a year earlier. He attributed the 1789 pandemic to a series of earthquakes in North America and to the eruption of Vesuvius on 29 October, which caused a darkness over Kentucky.

With pestilence sweeping across the world driven by a poisonous atmosphere, no form of quarantine was justified. But this was not the worst consequence of the *"erroneous system of specific contagion"* that the likes of Mead had forced upon mankind:

> *Had Mead, and other eminent physicians taken the same pains to lead mankind into truth, as into error, we should have long ago have introduced improvements into the arrangement and structure of our cities which would have secured our citizens from nine-tenths of the infectious diseases, by which they have always been alarmed and distressed.*

To prevent or mitigate pestilential diseases, Webster proposed specific public sanitation and personal hygiene measures, beginning with the cleaning of municipalities through the liberal use of water; the draining of marshes; proper design of wharves and docks; spacious lots with room for gardens; avoidance of excesses of diet, extreme exposure to the heat of the sun, and undue fatigue; and extensive bathing. By these means, local causes of pestilence are removed, and the body is strengthened to resist disease. If this fails, the only remedy is to *"remove (oneself) from the place where it exists."*

Yellow Fever in Philadelphia: 1793

> *Hot, dry winds forever blowing,*
> *Dead men to the grave-yards going:*
> *Constant hearses, Funeral verses;*
> *Oh! what plagues - there is no knowing!*
> *Priests retreating from their pulpits! -*
> *Some in hot, and some in cold fits*
> *In bad temper, Off they scamper,*
> *Leaving us - unhappy culprits!*
> *Doctors raving and disputing,*
> *Death's pale army still recruiting -*
> *What a pother One with t'other!*
> *Some a-writing, some a-shooting.*
> *Nature's poisons here collected,*
> *Water, earth, and air infected -*
> *O, what pity, Such a city,*
> *Was in such a place erected!*
> *Pestilence by Philip Freneau, Philadelphia 1793*

Such a place indeed! Hot and damp; no water system and only one sewer. Holes were dug to receive wastewater, dead animals and all kinds of noxious matters. South of the city lay swamps, marshes and stagnant water. All contributed to creating a most morbid atmosphere during summer time when the temperature was at its hottest and the air most heavy and foul. In 1793, with the exception of a few drops on 9 September and 12 October, no rain fell from 25 August to 15 October.

But Philadelphia was also the political, cultural and medical center of the United States. Following a century of extraordinary growth, that saw its' population grow from 5000 in 1720 to 30,000 on the eve of the Revolution, it was the center of the demand for independence and was America's capital from 1790 to 1800. Also, it was here where the first medical school had been established in 1765.

Politically, 1793 was a particularly turbulent year as thousands demonstrated to convince the Government of President Washington to enter the war between France and Great Britain on the side of the French. Also present were thousands of impoverished French refugees that had fled the revolution in Santo Domingo. In fact, the first arrivals were probably responsible for introducing yellow fever in Philadelphia in July. The outbreak of yellow fever led many to abandon the city thus probably sparing the nation a major political upheaval. It allowed Washington to not give his support to either side.

On 19 August 1793, in an alley on the waterfront of Philadelphia, Peter Aston died after a few days of illness. His physician was Benjamin Rush (1746-1813), who would lose another patient, Mary Shewell, on the same day. Rush soon learned from doctors who were treating Catherine LeMaigre, who was clearly dying of the same disease, that similar deaths had occurred on nearby streets. One of the doctors called Rush's attention to the stale, pungent smell in the air that came from rotting coffee that had been dumped on 24 July on a wharf only one block away. Rush seized upon this fact, seeing that it could explain the sudden outbreak of pestilential fever. In a letter to Dr John Redman, the President of the Fellows of the College of Physicians, he observed:

> *It should not surprise us, that this seed (coffee), so inoffensive in its natural state, should produce, after its putrefaction, a violent fever. The records of medicine furnish instances of similar fevers being produced, by the putrefaction of many other vegetable substances ... The rapid progress of the fever from Water Street, and the courses through which it travelled into other parts of the city, afford strong evidence that it was at first propagated chiefly by exhalation from the putrid coffee.*

These events shortly reminded Rush of the 1762 yellow fever in Philadelphia, which he had seen during his student days. He did not hesitate then to pronounce the disease the *bilious remitting yellow fever.*

Normally, the average August day in Philadelphia would see 3 to 5 burials; this number was quickly exceeded. By 24 August, it had risen to 17. Rush told the Mayor that the disease was carried by putrid miasmata in the air and advised him to clean up the city. The Governor asked Dr James Hutchinson, inspector of sickly vessels, for his opinion. The College of Physicians held a special meeting on 25 August to consider the best method of checking the progress of the disease. Sixteen of its 26 members showed up, including both Rush and Hutchinson. The day before, when Rush had learned that

Plague Legends

Hutchinson was denying the existence of any kind of pestilence, he wrote him, asserting that there really was a highly malignant fever, while hesitating to conclude if it was *"propagated by contagion, or by the original exhalation."* This time he withheld the diagnosis of yellow fever, only saying that the disease had all the symptoms of *"a mild remittent, and a typhus gravior."*

All members of the College agreed that there was a malignant fever abroad in the city. But as to its cause, they could not agree whether it was imported and contagious or domestic and carried by miasmatic air. One group believed it was contagious and had been introduced by the influx of Santo Dominicans, the other group, which included Rush, believed like all fevers, it arose from putrefied air. A committee was asked to prepare a report. Rush, a member, was asked to write it. On the 26th his report was considered and adopted unanimously. Rush avoided the words 'yellow fever', instead referring to the *"malignant and contagious fever, which now prevails."*

The report suggested eleven measures:

1. Avoid contact with any infected individuals;
2. Place a mark on houses where infected individuals reside;
3. Place infected persons "in the centre of large and airy rooms, in beds without curtains," and "pay the strictest regard to cleanliness, by frequently changing their body and bed linen, also by removing, as speedily as possible, all offensive matter from their rooms;"
4. Provide a large and airy hospital in the neighborhood of the city;
5. Stop tolling of bells;
6. Bury the dead in closed carriages as privately as possible;
7. Keep the streets and wharves as clean as possible - "as the contagion of the disease may be taken into the body and pass out of it, without producing the fever, unless it be rendered active by some occasional cause;" (which are addressed in the last 4 points)
8. Avoid all fatigue of body and mind;
9. Avoid standing or sitting in the sun, air currents or evening air;
10. Dress according to the weather;
11. Avoid intemperance and use fermented liquors, such as wine, beer, and cider, in moderation.

The report also noted that the College did not believe that fires were effective. They had reason *"to place more dependence upon the burning of gun-powder."*

After random gunshots had wounded several people, the mayor was shortly forced to forbid this as well.

Hutchinson gave his response on August 28. He asserted that a highly malignant fever was present, which was beginning to spread from its original location. He noted that the general opinion was that the "*contagion originated from some damaged coffee, or other putrefied vegetables and animal matters.*" However, since earlier cases had been reported some distance away from the docks, the coffee theory may not be correct. He did not think that it was an imported disease since he had "*learned of no foreigners or sailors that have hitherto been infected.*"

Meanwhile the public searched out its own remedies and came to their own conclusions concerning the origin of this terrible epidemic. Defoe's *The Plague Year* was read in search of advice. Rush had his own copy (a first edition), on which he made marginal notes and added observations.[38] Many, including women and small boys, took up smoking tobacco. Others placed their confidence in the chewing of garlic; some kept it in their pockets and shoes. Another popular method was to carry pieces of tarred rope in their hands or pockets and camphor bags tied around their necks. Most citizens probably believed that the Santo Dominicans had brought in the disease just as the earlier 1762 epidemic had been traced to the arrival of infected ships.

Once the epidemic became commonly known, citizens began to leave Philadelphia by any means they could find - carts, wagons, coaches, chairs, by horse or on foot. The United States Government essentially closed down. Similarly, Philadelphia's ability to administer began to fall apart as more and more city officials absented themselves from work. By the middle of September, mail delivery stopped, and only one newspaper was able to continue to publish on a regular basis. The mayor was forced to call for voluntary help to keep the business of the town going.

Rush, along with the other doctors that had not left, struggled to find a treatment that would work. He tried everything he could think of beginning with gentle purges, the prescription of various barks, and the application of blisters to the limbs, neck, and head. When this failed, he wrapped the sick in blankets saturated with warm vinegar, and tried to stimulate the liver by rubbing mercurial ointment on the patient's backside. He even tried pouring

---

[38] I have tried to locate Rush's copy of Defoe's book from historical libraries in Philadelphia but no-one has yet been able to find any record of it.

buckets of cold water over his patients. Then, in late August, he remembered having read an account of a yellow fever epidemic in Virginia in 1741 written by Dr John Mitchell. He searched and found Mitchell's paper and there he found words that struck him "*with the force of divine revelation.*"[39]

Mitchell believed that the disease was caused by an over-excitement of the body leading to the abdominal viscera being filled with blood. Thus its cure depended on depleting the body of all exciting stimuli and removing the excess blood. Bleeding and purging was the answer, even if the pulse was so thin you could hardly feel it. Rush increased the dosage that he had used to purge soldiers during the revolutionary war. His mercurial purge - ten grams each of calomel and jalap (the latter "*to carry the calomel through the bowels*") - became notorious as "*Rush's ten-and-ten.*" He instructed his disciples to repeat bleeding "*while the symptoms that first indicated it continue … until four-fifths of the blood contained in the body be drawn away.*" Fortunately he underestimated the amount of blood contained in the body; nevertheless, he was known to draw more than nine pints of blood from patients, an amount that is considered fatal.

With a sense of renewed confidence, Rush began a campaign to force this method upon his medical colleagues. He stopped physicians on the street to tell them about it. He informed the Fellows of the College of his cure and by 5 September, he was writing his wife that the pestilence was no more fatal than a common bilious fever. He even believed that his great purge and copious bleeding could prevent the disease.

An extraordinary meeting of the Fellows of the College of Physicians was called on 7 September to hear Redman speak on the nature and cure of the yellow fever of 1762. In it he reviewed the methods that had been tried then, methods that all were familiar with but which had not worked then nor were they working now. He did, however, observe with some hope the new system of treatment being used by Rush.

Rush published his cure so that he would not have to answer the many written requests that he received daily. It appeared on 11 September. By this time, he had already added five more grains of jalap to his regimen:

---

[39] Rush's religious convictions helped sustain him throughout the four months that the epidemic lasted during which time he tended to thousands of patients under the most horrifying and trying circumstances.

As soon as you feel pains in head or back, are nauseated or have chills and fever, take one of the powders (ten grains calomel, fifteen jalap) in a little sugar and water, every six hours, until they produce four or five large evacuations from the bowels. Drink plenty of water or gruel, lie abed and sweat. After the bowels are thoroughly cleansed, if the pulse be full and tense, be bled of eight or ten ounces from the arm, more, if tension continues. Light diet, fresh air, continuously open bowels, blisters on sides, neck and head, cleanliness above all, should be your regimen.

Rush was sure to be read since he was one of the most prominent citizens of Philadelphia. Not only was he one of the signatories of the Declaration of Independence, but he had helped organize the first anti-slavery society in America, had written extensively about the evils of drink and tobacco, and even helped Thomas Paine write his famous essay *Common Sense*.

The epidemic of 1762 had started in August and lasted into December. That of 1793 would also end with the coming of winter. Before its end, however, more than 5000 deaths were reported; the real number was no doubt considerably greater. More than 10% of Philadelphia's population had been lost in a matter of three months.

Rush largely failed to get his radical approach to treatment adopted by others. Instead, opposing methods were proposed and a war of letters and rumors began which would divide the medical community and embitter Rush for the rest of his life. He remained blind to the fact that his method simply did not work and may in fact have quickened the death or even caused the death of many. But Rush believed that he had prevented 6000 deaths that otherwise would have occurred. He occupied so important a place in American medicine that his so-called 'heroic therapeutics' would dominate medical practice in America for most of the 19th century.

Rush's Doctrine of the Unity of Fevers

The system of Dr Boerhaave long ago ceased to regulate the practice of physic. It was succeeded by the system of Dr Cullen... Dr Brown's system ... captivated a few young men for a while ... In the year 1790, (this) author ... promulgated some new principles in medicine suggested by the peculiar phaenomena of the disease of the United States. These new principles have been so much enlarged and improved by the successive observations and reasonings of many gentlemen in all the states, as to form a new system of medicine. This system rejects the nosological of diseases, and admits only of a single disease. (Rush)

Plague Legends

Herman Boerhaave (1668-1738) celebrated the name of Sydenham, calling *him* *"the shining light of England, that Apollo of the art."* Rush was known as America's Sydenham, yet when he came back from Edinburgh, which owed much of its fame to faculty members who had studied under Boerhaave and where Rush had obtained his medical degree in 1768, he proclaimed that his elder colleagues had been fools because they had followed Boerhaave.

To make matters even more complicated, it will be remembered that Sydenham was considered England's Hippocrates. Rush too was known as America's Hippocrates, but whereas both Sydenham and Boerhaave were respectful and admiring of that ancient healer, Rush condemned Hippocrates' reliance on the healing powers of nature, writing - *"It is impossible to calculate the mischief which Hippocrates has done by first marking Nature with his name and afterwards letting her loose on sick people."*

This all needs to be disentangled for it to make any sense, beginning with the importance of Boerhaave and working through the other influences on Rush (Cullen and Brown) to the point where Rush is standing on his own, admitting *"only of a single disease."*

Boerhaave was by far the most successful clinician and medical teacher of the 18th century. He made Leyden the medical center of the world in the course of the 37 years that he taught students from all of Europe and the New World. Boerhaave was a staunch defender of anatomy and assisted in many anatomical demonstrations and autopsies. He praised the work of Harvey and helped popularize that of Newton. He incorporated botany in his teachings, and he sponsored the great Linnaeus. Although critical of the iatrochemists, who, he argued, *"were miserably mistaken in general laws"* which they derived from *"their cant of elements, fictitious ferments, effervescences, antagonistic salts ...,"* this did not stop him from testing their theories experimentally and accepting chemistry as an essential part of physiology. It is perhaps in his role of bringing together all of the sciences in the teaching of medicine that he best deserves his fame.

Boerhaave pictured health in terms of a hydrostatic equilibrium, a balance of internal fluid pressures. He distinguished between disorders of the 'solids' and those of the 'blood and humors'. While generally favoring a mechanical view of the body, Boerhaave was critical of Cartesian mechanists who based their beliefs more on analogy than on observations. For him, they were too eager to imagine that living organisms act as inanimate objects do.

Boerhaave's admiration of Sydenham rested on their mutual respect for the Hippocratic tradition of bedside teaching, the taking of careful case histories from their patients, and relying on the curative power of nature. They shared similar concepts of disease, both noting their seasonality and their tendency to attack those who today are known as high-risk individuals. Also, they practiced a relatively mild form of treatment with much reliance on small doses of medicine, exercise, fresh air and changes in diet.

Fevers occupied a far less important place in Boerhaave's system than it did among his followers. He concluded that a rapid pulse was the one feature by which a physician could judge a fever to be present. Given how important fevers were to Cullen, John Brown (1722-87) and Rush, it is perhaps this more than any other fact that led them to seek alternative systems, ones in which fevers featured prominently. Cullen and Brown were leading faculty members when Rush was at Edinburgh. Brown initially was an assistant to Cullen but after he broke from Cullen he began to give lectures on his own system.

Cullen, like Boerhaave, appreciated the value of chemistry and wrote extensively on all aspects of medical practice. But he rejected Boerhaave's emphasis on the blood vessels and their contents as the major source of disease, replacing these simple mechanical explanations with the 'vital' activity of the nervous system. For Cullen, almost all diseases were 'neurotic' in the sense that disease disturbed the normal functioning of the nervous system. He labeled the disordered action of the nervous system a 'spasm' - earning him the nickname 'Old Spasm'.

Pyrexia (all fevers) dominated Cullen's disease classification. He separated essential fevers from symptomatic fevers, developing a system consisting of five orders - fevers, i.e. those pyrexia which lacked any other major symptom (e.g. 'typhus'), inflammations (e.g. hepatitis), eruptions (e.g. plague), hemorrhages (e.g. consumption) and fluxes (e.g. dysentery). Thus, Cullen placed most infectious diseases in one of the fever categories.

Cullen's view on causation and treatment was rather complex. Many factors could cause fevers, e.g., contagious atmospheric matter that arose from the bodies of the sick (human effluvia), miasmas that arose from marshes and standing water (marsh effluvia), heat, cold, fear, and dirt. However, he believed the same external factors could cause different diseases in different individuals, depending on the state of their nervous system. Thus, treatment depended on external as well as internal factors. Cullen's therapeutic advice, however, was not firmly defined, although he believed in an energetic intervention, one that did not rely on the healing powers of nature. No doubt, it was this characteristic of Cullen's theory that was particularly attractive to Rush, at the time he was trying to replace Boerhaave's teaching with that of Cullen.

Cullen believed that most external causes, for example those of contagion or miasma, exerted a sedative influence on the body, inducing debility. A debilitated state demanded supportive therapy to restore vigor - wine, tonics, and cinchona bark. He did not favor bloodletting, although this and other antiphlogistic remedies had a place, especially in warm climates. It is probably due to this position that caused Rush to later turn against Cullen as well.

Brown, known by some as the Scottish Paracelsus, took Cullen's ideas to the extreme. Having determined that 'excitability' was the central property of all living things, an excess ('sthenic' condition) or deficiency ('asthenic' condition) of this property gave rise to sickness. Brown believed that most illness resulted from the exhaustion of 'excitability' and thus must be treated by stimulants, of which spirits, wine, and opium were deemed the most useful. For Brown, physicians erroneously justified the giving of a specific drug for each specific disease by the presence of a multiplicity of causes. Having reduced the cause of disease to a variation in the degree of excitement, it logically followed that treatment needed to excite or to debilitate. Following his own treatment for gout, he became heavily addicted to both alcohol and opium.

Some historians have suggested that at the time Rush was studying at Edinburgh, the school was heavily under the influence of certain philosophical principles as expounded by such thinkers as David Hume (1711-1776) and Adam Smith (1723-1790). They, like Newton, believed in seeking the simplest causes for the important phenomena of life. To what degree Rush fell under their influence is probably not known. Nevertheless, like Brown, his advice took on a simplistic character, whether it was in the practice of medicine or in the many other spheres of life that he energetically contributed to.

Upon his return from Europe in 1769, Rush attacked his fellow colleagues who still believed in Boerhaave's theories because he had come to accept Cullen's position on the importance of fevers. In time, however, for reasons indicated above, he took Cullen to task too. Another reason for Rush's shifting of position was that he had come to believe that American diseases were peculiar to it. America's climate, environment, diet and living habits were different from those of Europe, so in accordance with Hippocrates, it followed that its diseases were different as well. At the same time, he argued, like Sydenham, that diseases changed in time and space. This led him to conclude that efforts to classify them were useless and would retard medical progress.

Rush in 1804 explained to an English correspondent - "*The extremes of heat and cold produc(e) greater extremes of violence in our fevers than in yours.*" He was referring to 'his' malaria and yellow fever, while his correspondent probably had fevers due to typhus, tuberculosis, malaria and several other diseases in mind.[40] Confusing the matter even further was the long-held belief that individual patients could exhibit different fevers during the course of the same illness. In mid-19th century, for example, physicians still spoke of how "*neglected or maltreated*" malarial fevers could become "*classic yellow fever.*" This followed logically from the basic idea that a disease was an effect caused by multiple factors. As those factors changed, so would the disease.

It is possible that Rush was influenced by the work of Georges Louis Leclerc, Comte de Buffon (1701-1788), one of Europe's leading naturalists, who argued that the New World had been created after the rest of the world so that nothing there had reached its full growth potential. This, in combination with the scarcity of human life there, had led the atmosphere to be particularly contaminated thus causing deadly diseases. Also, Hippocrates' text on *Air, Waters and Places,* having recently become available in English, French and German, was being restudied, and other investigators were realizing that what Hippocrates had written applied only to Thrace and Thessaly in the 4th century BC; each region of the world needed to observe its own conditions and diseases and arrive at its own correlations.

---

[40] The English author Frederick Marryat (1792-1848) would later rely on Rush's views concerning America's extreme climatic "*excitement*" to characterise its diseases as being primarily neurological, taking such forms as *tic douloureux* or *delirium tremens.* He "*unhesitatingly pronounced (America's) climate to be bad, being injurious to them in the two important points, of healthy vigour in the body and healthy action of the mind, enervating the one and tending to demoralize the other.*"

DEFENCE OF BLOOD-LETTING

BLOOD-LETTING, as a remedy for fevers, and certain other diseases, having lately been the subject of much discussion, and many objections having been made to it, which appear to be founded in error and fear, I have considered that a defence of it, by removing those objections, might render it more generally useful, in every part of the United States.

I shall begin this subject by remarking, that blood-letting is indicated, in fevers of great morbid excitement,

1. by the sudden suppression or dimunition of the natural discharges by the pores, bowels, and kidneys, whereby a plethora is induced in the system.

For Rush yellow fever was "*a monarchical disorder.*" It was at the apex of the fevers with "*the common bilious remitting fever*" being next and the "*intermitting fever*" last. They were "*only different grades of the same disease.*" To believe otherwise, he argued, would be to resemble the Indian or African savage "*who considers water, dew, ice, frost, and snow, as distinct essences.*"[41] All fevers depended on a single cause, namely - "*a morbid action in the blood vessels,*" whose action could vary in force, frequency, or locus of its activity. Having reduced fevers to 'one', he declared that he had cut *materia medica* to fifteen or twenty drugs, and made medicine "*a science so simple that two year's study instead of four or more were sufficient.*"

Rush died in 1813 of typhus during an epidemic that had spread from Europe to the United States. True to his beliefs, he insisted on being bled even though his physicians felt he was too weak and that bleeding would be dangerous. Some thought at the time that bleeding hastened his death. This may have been the case since had he not united the fevers into one he might have learned, what others had already learned, namely that typhus is a fever best left unbled. In the middle of the 18th century, in England, mortality was lowest wherever there was a shortage of doctors, i.e., where there was less bleeding. Later in the 19th century, George B. Wood, Professor of the Theory and Practice of Medicine in the University of Pennsylvania and President of the College of Physicians of Philadelphia, would state that bleeding "*genuine typhus ... is often capable of doing much harm, and death has frequently been the result of its injudicious use.*"

---

[41] Charles Caldwell, a student at the University of Pennsylvania in the 1790s, in his graduating thesis, followed Rush in advocating "*the original sameness*" of water on the brain, membranous croup (diphtheria), and infantile diarrhea!

Rush is considered by many to have been the best physician in America at the end of the 18ᵗʰ century. He was one of the 400 out of around 3500 physicians who had a medical degree. He said of himself that *"Medicine is my wife and Science my mistress,"* which later led Oliver Wendell Holmes (1809-1894) to caustically comment, *"I do not think that the breach of the Seventh Commandment can be shown to have been an advantage to the legitimate owner of his affections."*

Webster's Views on the Origin of Yellow Fever

True it is, the sudden deaths of a few persons yearly makes no public noise; even if the disease is ever so malignant. While it does not threaten to become epidemic, it creates no alarm. But when some peculiarity of season or contagion spreads the disorder over a whole city, then it becomes an object of notice, and all the world is anxious to know where it originates. (Webster)

Webster met and corresponded with Benjamin Franklin, George Washington and other leading minds, including Rush, when he was a relatively young man. His campaign to 'reform' the American language attracted these revolutionary leaders; Webster even contemplated at one point becoming the private secretary of Washington, but rejected it when he realised how much that would interfere with his own intellectual activity.

By the late 1780's, he and Rush were in active correspondence, initially over his plans to found a literary and political magazine in Philadelphia. As noted earlier, the influenza epidemic of 1789 and 1790 attracted his interest, and being a keen observer of natural phenomena, he added disease outbreaks to his diary recordings of temperatures, precipitation, and the character of the prevailing winds. Relying on information that he obtained in libraries and from correspondence with physicians throughout America, he accumulated the basic facts for his 1799 *History of Epidemic and Pestilential Diseases,* discussed earlier.

In keeping with Rush's *"unity of fevers,"* Webster did not differentiate one epidemic disease from another. He determined from the description of plague at Athens by Thucydides that it and yellow fever *"are the same."* The distemper that struck New England in the early part of the 18ᵗʰ century, he considered to be the *"plague among children."* He believed that there was a natural progression from one plague species to another and that their seriousness increased over time, e.g. measles and influenza gradually progressed to throat or angina distempers and finally to pestilential fever.[42]

Climate was the critical factor that determined when and among what population, epidemics would break out. Webster was struck by the fact that visitors to a new climate were always more prone to illness than were the indigenous population. He claimed, for example, that *"one half of the northern gentlemen, of my acquaintance who have attempted establishments in the southern states, have died within the first or second year."* That they fell ill in America was also of importance in that it convinced him that all diseases were present in the states, one need not search in foreign lands for their origin.

In a series of 25 long and detailed public letters addressed to Doctor William Currie, written in a two-month period at the end of 1797, Webster further developed his ideas. Currie, who was an eminent Philadelphian physician, had undertaken to inform the public regarding the nature and origin of the 1797 outbreak of yellow fever. Rush had already informed Webster that *"Currie is now the oracle of our city upon the subject of yellow fever."* In fact, Rush acknowledged to Webster that Curries' letters *"have made a greater impression upon our citizens than any thing that has ever been published in Philadelphia upon the subject."* He encouraged Webster to continue his letters and to preserve them in the form of a pamphlet *"for the benefit of all the States in the Union and of posterity."* To which he added:

> I consider you as my advocate ...

Rush was hoping to win in 1797 the battle that he had lost in 1793 to prove that yellow fever was a local disease. During the closing days of the earlier epidemic, when the Governor had asked the College of Physicians for an

---

[42] A.A. Milne captured this idea in his poem *Sneezle,* in which Christopher Robin is sick with wheezles and sneezles. When famous physicians arrive, they note the state of his throat and ask if he suffered from thirst, and then go on:

> They asked if the sneezles
> Came *after* the wheezles,
> Or if the first sneezle
> Came first.
> They said, "If you teazle
> A sneezle
> Or wheezle,
> A measle
> May easily grow.

account of the cause of the pestilence, the *"foreign origin"* faction had won. Rush, appalled at this *"conspiracy"* against him resigned from that body, taking the opportunity to send the College a copy of Sydenham's work. Four years later, he was still attempting to organize physicians who believe in *"the domestic origin of the yellow fever."* With the help of Webster he was able to generate enough interest to eventually help establish such a group. This group would offer one of the few instances when early American medicine influenced thinking on the Continent, as discussed in the next Chapter, when Europe was threatened by yellow fever.

Currie discussed and rejected the previous belief that the 1793 epidemic had originated in the West Indies. He now believed that it had come from the island of Boullam, on the Coast of Africa. Starting from there, it had been carried by ship to Grenada, from whence it was communicated to other islands and eventually the United States.[43] Webster tracked down all the information that he could find concerning Boullam and its links with the West Indies and arrived at totally opposing conclusions.

He learned that a settlement of around 300 people from England had been established on Boullam for the purpose of cultivating cotton for the Manchester market. They suffered much illness on the way there, after they arrived and on subsequent voyages, including those to the West Indies. Webster was able to explain each outbreak in terms of exposure to changing climatic conditions. No new imported disease was evident at any point of the communication routes involved. In fact, he determined that it was *"fanatic enthusiasm for the abolition of the slave trade"* that had led to the deliberate plot to show that the African coast was infected with pestilence! Although he found the slave trade *"nefarious,"* he was deeply shocked that a *"false theory of specific contagion"* could be thus propagated:

> *Where is the epithet that will express the baseness of the undertaking, or describe the melancholy effects of the principle? Surely, Sir, men have not thus a right to trifle with the truth, and with social confidence and happiness.*

The example of Boullam was but one of many examples used by Webster to disprove specific instances where a foreign origin was hypothesized. In the

---

[43] In Currie, Webster was dealing with a very knowledgeable opponent, Currie having himself written in 1792 *An Historical Account of the Climates and Diseases of the United States of America.*

course of his studies he found it necessary, as befitting a lexicographer, to define more carefully what was meant by the terms *infection* and *contagion*, words that *"in ordinary language ... are ... synonimous (sic)..."* - *Infection* derives from *inficio*, which signifies *"conveyance from one thing to another by introduction, infusion or contact"* while *contagion* comes from *contingo*, which is *"something communicated by touch."* By *contagious* disease, he meant *"one which may be and usually is communicated from person to person, by the touch or near approach, independent of season or accidental circumstances; as the small pox, measles and hooping-cough."*

An *infectious* disease, on the other hand, he considered to be *"one capable of being received from diseased persons only under certain circumstance"* such as crowded population, hot weather, close rooms, as demonstrated by the *"malignant yellow fever or plague."* Particularly important was a changing climate. Webster's review of past epidemics in the world convinced him that both these diseases seldom affected *"the natives of Africa and the West Indies,"* while those who live in *"temperate climates, which experience alternatively great heat and extreme cold, are precisely those which have most to fear from the plague, or yellow fever."* Since both diseases were infectious, and arose from changing conditions of the climate, it followed that quarantine measures were not required for either; instead, both could be prevented by cleaning up the environment along the lines described earlier for influenza.

Webster, an avowed and firm *"believer the being and perfections of a God,"* did not believe that *"that being ever did or will interpose a miraculous power to change the laws of nature and prevent disease, in places where its natural causes exist."* It remains for man, not *"the almighty power (to) cleanse dirty streets and cellars"* and to save those *"who wallow in filth, intemperance and debauchery, from falling victims to fever."*

Webster recognized two kinds of epidemical constitutions - partial or local, and general. Almost all of the outbreaks discussed in his letters to Currie provided examples of the local constitution at work. It is in his 1799 publication where one learns of the natural phenomena that account for a general epidemical constitution, e.g. earthquakes, volcanic explosions and comets, as described earlier in his analysis of the global movement of influenza. Rush wrote of these in 1798:

> *You have opened a mine of precious metals to the lovers of science and friends of humanity. I have for some time past suspected that the malignant constitution of the atmosphere taken notice by Hippocrates and Dr.*

*Sydenham pervaded our **whole** globe, at the **same** time and that it was somehow produced by the influence of some part, or parts of the solar system upon our earth. But you have demonstrated that to be true which was only a floating idea in my mind...*

Currie dismissed the work, commenting that it is *"as much the creature of the imagination as the tales of the fairies."*

* * * * *

At the end of the 17th century, Boyle, Sydenham and others had proposed a systematic effort to link disease with various environmental factors, particularly those associated with the weather. Here and there individual investigators dutifully recorded and published their findings but by and large little if anything came of their efforts. Only in France, in the 1770s, was there a short-lived initiative to create a 'medicine of epidemics', one, however, that did not survive the medical reforms undertaken during the revolution. Instead of developing in an organized, institutional manner, the study of epidemics remained isolated, individual affairs, such as the one undertaken by Webster at the close of the century.

Rush, Webster and others made observations that were shouting to be interpreted 'correctly', that is, with the realization that the infectious diseases, such as plague, yellow fever and malaria, were caused by the bite of some small insect whose presence was dictated by seasonal and climatic factors.[44] Rush had noted, for example, that *"morbid exhalations"* associated with the effluvia of millponds *"produce fevers at the distance of two to three miles, where they are not opposed by houses, woods, or a hilly country."* Rush's most striking observations concerned what today we know to be malarial fevers, and his findings correspond well with what is known about the malaria-carrying *Anopheles* mosquito. Webster had occasion to study the sites where yellow fever outbreaks occurred and noted how these invariably were quarters where filth had accumulated, i.e. sites today known to be favored by the *Aedes aegypti* mosquito.

---

[44] In France during 1781-2 influenza pandemic it was conjectured for a while that the air had become infected from the far greater than normal number of insects in the air known as 'la grippe', thus giving rise to that name for this disease. Emmanuel Kant (1724-1804) speculated that noxious insects had made their way from China via Russia. Thus, the idea of insects being responsible for disease was not out of the question at that time.

Plague Legends

The line of study initiated in America by Rush and Webster would continue (see malaria discussion in Chapter VI) but, for the immediate future, the radical medical reforms that had taken place in France dominated medical advance, as discussed next.

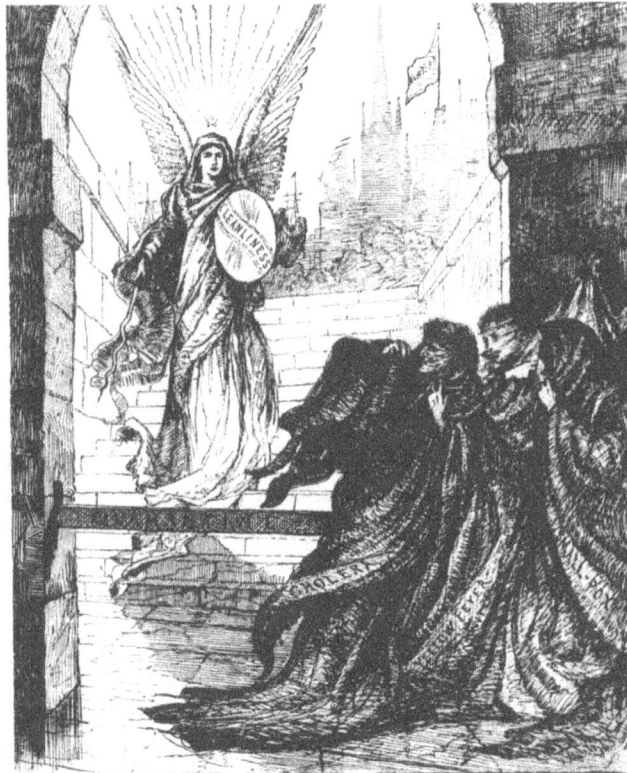

AT THE GATES.
Our safety depends upon official vigilance.

VI

19th Century - Recognition of Disease Specificity

Opens the Door to Specific Disease Causation

At the end of the 18th century there were physicians who, following de Sauvages, believed in the existence of literally thousands of diseases. On the other extreme, there was Rush and his followers who rejected the notion of distinct febrile diseases and united the fevers into one group. At issue, however, was not simply the question of 'how many' diseases there were, since the very notion of specificity was not commonly accepted. Furthermore, even where disease specificity was accepted, it did not mean that one was any closer to understanding the etiology of any particular disease. As late as 1882, August Hirsch, a German medical historian, put the problem in these terms for influenza:

> *Influenza is a specific infective disease like cholera, typhoid, smallpox, and others, and it has at all times and in all places borne a stamp of uniformity in its configuration and in its course such as almost no other infective disease has. Its genesis presupposes, therefore, a uniform and specific cause ... There can be no objection to calling this specific cause by the name of "miasma," so long as we remember that nothing more is expressed thereby than that which the physicians of the 16th and 17th centuries called a "fouling of the air," and that, in setting up a name in the place of an obscure conception, we do not bring ourselves by that means a single step nearer to a knowledge of the cause of the disease.*

How specificity of disease gained the upper hand is the story of the first part of the 19th century. Disease etiology as such only began to be resolved towards the very end of the century. Intriguingly, from the historical point of view, was the continuity of Rush's reductionism in that of Broussais, a French physician who gave birth to equally simplistic and erroneous theories concerning fevers around the time of Rush's death. Nevertheless, the belief in disease specificity did emerge, albeit slowly. The recognition of microbes as a necessary feature of each etiological story took the whole century to unfold. For some, the search for the disease-causing agents and their so-called modes of transmission lasted well into the 20th century.

Broussais Uses Pathological Anatomy to Show All Fevers to Be the Same

Several autopsies will give you more light than twenty years of observation of symptoms. (Bichat)

If corpses have sometimes seemed to be silent, it is because we were ignorant of the art of questioning them. (Broussais)

Galen had suggested - "*There are very few essential symptoms of disease which do not point to the affected part,*" and Harvey had noted - "*The examination of a single body of one who has died of consumption or some other disease of long-standing, is of more service to medicine than the dissection of ten men who have been hanged.*" But neither Galen nor Harvey pursued these expressed ideas. Others did, however, and slowly over the centuries their results appeared, but in a fragmented and isolated manner. In 1679, Theophilus Bonetus, a Swiss physician, compiled almost three thousand of these cases, drawn from 470 authors. Unfortunately, the published compilation was very badly organized and lacked a useful index. The importance of this publication lay in the fact that it convinced Giovanni Battista Morgagni (1682-1771), who read it at a young age, "*to supply the deficiencies ... in the Sepulchretum* (the title of Bonetus' work) *... (and) to reform the indexes.*" Morgagni devoted much of his professional career to this effort.

Not all physicians at that time believed in the value of dissection. The famous name of Sydenham, for example, is not to be found among Bonetus' 470 authors. Sydenham never practiced any dissection, rejecting them as useless. He alone of all the doctors who attended in July 1680 the fatally ill Lord Ossory did not participate in the post-mortem examination. Furthermore, he opposed the teaching of botany and anatomy - "*Anatomy - Botany - Nonsense*" he told a student. He knew of an old woman "*who understands botany better, and as for anatomy, my butcher can dissect a joint full and well ... you must go to the bedside, it is there alone you can learn disease.*" Nevertheless, he was not as extreme as Locke who believed that - "*Though we cut into the inside, we see but the outside of things and make out new superfices to stare at ... Nature performs all her operations in the body by parts so minute and insensible that I think nobody will ever hope to come to a sight of them.*" Sydenham allowed that when anatomists can understand the inner workings of the 'animalculum', then he was ready to believe that - "*he will be able to show the very operations of those parts in man, and till he does that he does very little towards the discovery of the cause and cure of diseases.*"

Opponents to dissection also included those who recognized the futility of dissections whose only aim was to confirm Galen's anatomy. Such a picture was portrayed by La Mettrie (1709-1753) in his satirical criticism of medicine as practiced by Parisian doctors in the 1740s. Surgeons did the cutting while physicians read from the *"venerable texts of Hippocrates and Galen."* In one of his more aggressive stage pieces, one character says of doctors - *"I regard a physician, even one of the best, as a machine which when tapped always resonates Hippocrates or Galen and never makes another sound."* It was almost the same picture that Vesalius had drawn some 200 hundred years earlier.

Morgagni, like Vesalius, benefited from the more advanced development of medicine in Italy. He started keeping careful account of pre- and post-mortem results while he was a medical assistant in Bologna (1701-1707). Over the next fifty years he accumulated some seven hundred case histories. These took the form of seventy letters written to a young man, and were arranged according to 1. Diseases of the Head, 2. Diseases of the Thorax, 3. Diseases of the Belly, 4. Surgical and Universal Disorders, and 5. Supplement. Each case history is several pages long; the total work, which he did not publish until 1761, is twenty-four hundred pages. Its title is *De Sedibus et Causis Morborum per Anatomen Indagatis* (*De Sedibus* for short), or in English, *The Seats and Causes of Disease Investigated by Anatomy*. By combining excellent clinical and anatomical skills, he was able to correlate clinical with anatomical findings better than any of his predecessors had.

Although Morgagni's work is considered the beginning of the modern age of pathology, remnants of *Hippocratic* and *Galenic* traditions remained. Following Hippocrates, his rich and detailed observations and records included the patients diet, condition in life, and manner of employment. Like *Galen* he considered the *"quantity or state of the blood or other humors."*

The next great advance in the development of an anatomical conception of disease took place towards the end of the century when Parisian hospitals were turned into institutions that facilitated the investigation of disease. Pathological findings during autopsy were checked against bedside diagnosis and the clinical course of different diseases. It was dubbed the 'anatomic-pathological approach'; it brought together surgical with medical training, and in a short period of time made Paris the world's center for medical training. The history of this revolution is rich and complex.

In the year that Morgagni died, Marie Francois Xavier Bichat (1771-1802) was born at Thoirette, France. He was one of the founders of the French School at

Paris which became a leading medical school during the early part of the 19th century. In 1800 he published *Traité des Membranes* and in 1801 *Anatomie Générale Appliquée a la Physiologie et a la Médicine*. He died the following year of a severe fever in the thirty-first year of his life. Bichat could accomplish as much as he did in such a short period largely due to the incredible effort made during the French revolution to 'modernize' medical education, i.e. to bring together anatomy and pathology within the context of large teaching hospitals. Only in this way was it possible for Bichat to perform more than 600 autopsies in a period of 12 months.

Bichat viewed organs and their systems as made up of sheets of protoplasm called tissues. His *Anotomie* distinguishes twenty-one basic structures, most of which were one form of tissue or another, e.g. the tissue of the exhaling vessels, that of the absorbents, medullar tissue, fibrous tissue, fibro-cartilaginous tissue, animal muscular tissue, mucous membrane, serous membrane, and synovial membrane. He described and classified tissues not only according to their organization, but also to their functions, vital powers and sympathies. Instead of referring simply to inflammation of the heart, he wrote of pericarditis, myocarditis, endocarditis, i.e. inflammation of the outer, middle and inner tissues surrounding the heart.

Bichat taught that similar tissue in different organs and parts of the body can be expected to suffer similar degeneration when it is diseased; thus, "*whatever may be the place in which the serous membranes are found, their diseases are analogous,*" and, "*the cutaneous system is the exclusive seat of certain morbid affections, such as tetter, syphilis, eruptions, and inflammatory pustules.*" He believed that a lasting classification of disease would be one that reflected the different nature of the different tissues and membranes in the body - "*since diseases are only alterations of the vital properties, and each texture differs from the others in its properties...*" Although he discussed therapeutics, Bichat did not offer any particular method of treatment beyond the choice of remedies according to John Brown's classification into sthenic and asthenic remedies, i.e. depressants and stimulants.

Francois Joseph Victor Broussais (1772-1838), a former Napoleonic soldier, came to Paris in 1799 to complete his medical studies. There he fell under the influence of Bichat and joined the group of physicians in Paris practicing the new anatomic-pathological approach. After receiving his degree in 1803 he became a military doctor with the imperial armies of Napoleon, eventually rising to the position of inspecteur général of the military medical corps. This position gave him considerable power, prestige and time to pursue his studies of fevers. He was one of the first members of the Académie de Médecine founded in 1823.

In 1808 Broussais published his *Histoire des phlegmasies ou inflammations chroniques fondée sur de nouvelles observations de clinique et d'anatomie pathologique,* in which he returned to an ancient idea that fever and inflammation are pathologically related. Following his teacher Bichat, inflammation of the tissues took precedence over other pathological forms. However, contrary to his predecessors, he regarded local lesions as the **cause** of symptoms, representing as they did *"the cry of the suffering organ."* He accused his predecessor's as having created arbitrary disease entities. He questioned the disease classification that had so dominated the second half of the previous century. In 1861 Armand Trousseau (1801-1867) would say of him:

> *Thirty to forty years ago, we seemed to have quite lost sight of the traditions of past centuries. Broussais had made a tabula rasa of everything said prior to his day, and pretended to have reestablished medicine on new foundations ...*

Like his mentors, Broussais examined corpses to find evidence of revealing tissue damage. Influenced by his numerous dissections of cases of typhoid fever (see next section), he ended up limiting his pathology to lesions of the gastro-intestinal tract. Once focussed there, and with the aid of newly invented scissors that readily exposed the intestines in their entirety, he was able to find these lesions in all autopsies. From this he concluded that all febrile diseases involved a chemical reaction to excessive stimuli, the inflammation being transmitted along the gastrointestinal mucosa. It was, he wrote, *"the destiny of the stomach always to be irritated."*

In 1816 he announced - *"All classifications that tend to make us regard disease as particular beings are defective ..."* In a publication of 1824 he systematically outlined how each fever previously thought to be a different disease was in fact but one manifestation of the same irritation. Thus, to take an extreme example, malaria was a periodic gastro-entiritis.

Broussais had established, so he thought, a morphological basis for Brown's clinical differentiation between sthenic and asthenic cases. Like Brown he grossly oversimplified therapeutics. Since 97% of patients were sthenic they needed treatment which diminished their *"excitability."*[45] For this he settled almost exclusively on treatment by bloodletting (by means of leaches) and a starvation diet. He prescribed 60, 80, 100 leaches at the same time, 250 in one day, and 800 in the course of treating the same clinical episode. In 1825 alone, the Hôtel-Dieu used more than 600,000 of them. Under his influence, the demand for leeches was so great that the supply in France became exhausted! Their importation rose from two or three million to 41.5 million per year.[46] And bleeding was not confined to fevers; it was used for constitutional diseases as well.[47]

Broussais did not lack critics. To the end of his life, he was the object of passionate attack. René Laënnec (1781-1826), the inventor of the stethoscope, and Pierre Louis (1787-1872), the inventor of the numerical method of clinical statistics, were particularly opposed to his theories. But neither Laënnec nor Louis had the ears of their students at the time. Students flocked to hear Broussais lecture while Louis never occupied a professorial chair. From 1816 onwards Broussais' thinking attracted an immense following, one that was not confined to France. Only in the 1830s did his star begin to decline. Holmes, who was a medical student of Louis in Paris during the period 1833-35, and who played a major role in introducing the new French ideas and methodology into the United States, said of him:

> *Broussais was in those days like an old volcano which has pretty nearly used up its fire and brimstone, but is still boiling and bubbling in its*

---

[45] Brown believed that 97% of patients owed their illnesses to asthenia and required stimulation. Later, in the beginning of the 19th century, English doctors turned to bleeding fevers, perhaps under the influence of Broussais as well as Rush, or, as suggested by several historians, because the disease pattern of England had changed.

[46] Although leeches take us a bit outside the main subject of this book, I cannot help note that much of the preface to the fifth edition of Wood's *Practice of Medicine*, published in 1858, concerns this subject. Earlier editions had not noted that American leeches draw at most only one-fourth as much blood as the European. The number prescribed in the text presumes the use of American stock. Thus, anyone wishing to employ European leeches, *"should employ not more than one for every four directed."* One cannot help but wonder how many patients had been bled by the use of European leeches following the earlier editions of this publication!

[47] Pasteur suffered a severe cerebral haemorrhage in October 1868. One of his attending physicians, Dr Andral, applied 16 leeches behind his ears and from the next day his speech improved and his recovery, which would take several months, began. It was the use of leeches, says a 1931 French scientific publication, that saved Pasteur's life.

*interior and now and then sends up a spirt of lava and volley of pebbles. His theories of irritation and inflammation as the cause of disease, and the practice which sprang from them, ran over the fields of medicine like flame over the grass of the prairies. The way in which that knotty-featured, savage old man would bring out the word **irritation** with rattling and rolling reduplication of the resonant letter **r** - might have taught a lesson in articulation to Salvani. But Broussais' theories languished and well-nigh became obsolete, and this no doubt added vehemence to his defence of his cherished dogmas.*

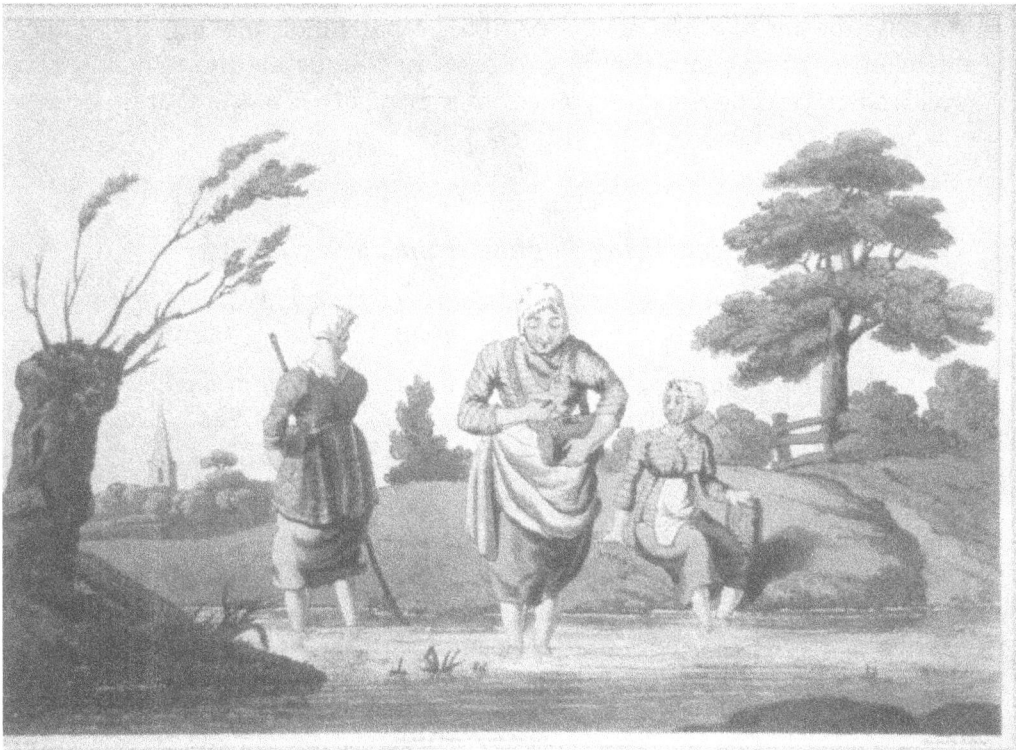

Despite Holmes' judgement, we find in Trousseau's *Clinique Médicale de L'Hotel-dieu de Paris* (2nd edit), published in 1865, an indication that the 'doctrines' of Broussais (and Brown) concerning the (non)existence of specific diseases were still influencing medical ideas and language. In Germany, where Broussais' teaching had an enormous vogue, the doctrine of specificity was disregarded up to the time of Pasteur and Koch.[48] And, although anecdotal in nature, the following excerpt from George Elliot's novel Middlemarch published in 1874 indicates that Broussais' influence was still felt more than 40 years after his death:

Oh, Lydgate ... I think he is likely to be first rate - has studied in Paris, knew Broussais; has ideas, you know - wants to raise the profession.[49]

This scene is situated around 1830. Lydgate eventually gives up trying to reform the practice of local rural doctors in Middlemarch and achieves some clinical fame in London before he died at the age of fifty of diphtheria, probably during the pandemic of 1855. Was Elliot making an ironical statement in having him die of a disease that Broussais thought not to be specific? This can't be ruled out, since other medical aspects of that time are so well presented in her work.

Distinguishing Typhus from Typhoid Fever

We should conjecture that the two diseases are widely and entirely different in symptoms, anatomical characters, treatment, and mode of transmission.

It affords us, then, great advantages in the investigation of the history of fevers, to begin with the typhoid, as the best known of these affections. (Gerhard)

Louis gave typhoid fever its name in an 1829 publication in which he had compiled masses of data concerning its anatomy, pathology and therapy. This name covered fevers that others, earlier, had designated putrid, gastro-enteritis, adynamic, ataxique, among others. He compared the postmortem findings of 50 patients who had died of a particular form of fever with 83 controls who had died from other causes. Those who had 'typhoid' exhibited

---

[48] Hans Zinsser points out that as late as 1878, when Koch published his treatise on the etiology of wound infection, specificity was not generally accepted, and the supposed metamorphosis of bacterial species had first to be scientifically refuted by Cohn, Koch and their pupils before it could be assumed that a given infectious disease was always the result of infection with a definite and constant species of bacteria.

[49] To which the listener replies: *Hang it, do you think that is quite sound? - upsetting the old treatment, which has made Englishmen what they are?*

particular forms of lesions in the intestinal tract. Louis used the term 'typhoid' because he believed that it was strongly related to typhus fever.

Louis was not the first to uncover the specific lesions produced by typhoid. Willis, as noted in Chapter IV, had done so in middle of the 17th century. In 1813 Marc-Antoine Petit (1762-1840) and Étienne-Renaud-Augustin Serres (1786-1868) published a monograph on entero-mesenteric fevers following an epidemic that had attacked Paris the preceding two years. Shortly thereafter, Pierre-Fidèle Bretonneau (1778-1862) described the clinical patterns and intestinal lesions following an epidemic in Tours. He gave the name *dothienentérite* to this disease, a neologism derived from two Greek words to mean abscess in the intestine.

Bretonneau's work on typhoid fever was written up between 1821 and 1827 but not published until 1922. In this work he attacked Broussais' doctrine of gastro-entiritis, stating that he never found a trace of gastritis in numerous autopsies of (non-typhoid) fever that he had performed. Despite the work of Louis, Petit, Serres and Bretonneau, however, typhus, typhoid and many other fevers remained one disease in the minds of many, especially the followers of Broussais.

Slowly evidence began to accumulate that allowed typhus to be distinguished from typhoid. This was important since there were many situations where only one of the two diseases was present. As early as the 1816-19 typhus epidemic in Edinburgh, pathologists were not able to find any lesions in typhus cases. This was to be more definitely shown by William Wood Gerhard (1809-1872) who was able to study a typhus epidemic that struck Philadelphia in 1836.

Gerhard (quoted above) was in the ideal position to demonstrate how the two diseases differed. After having received his diploma from the University of Pennsylvania in 1832 he went abroad for 2 years to continue his studies with Louis in Paris. There he had first hand experience with typhoid, a disease so frequent in Paris as to be *"almost the only fever which can be said to be endemic there."*

Upon his return to Philadelphia he initiated studies along the lines of Louis and demonstrated the presence of typhoid there, *"although less common than at Paris."* He noted that those suffering from typhoid fever had recently had *"an abrupt change of food and habits of life,"* somewhat along the lines that Webster had used to characterize an 'infectious' disease. He examined the pathological consequences of remittent and intermittent fevers and found internal "*morbid conditions*" but dissimilar to those caused by typhoid.

Then in the winter of 1835-36 a form of fever appeared "*not commonly met with at the hospitals.*" In March 1836 admissions were more numerous and "*attracted greater attention from their occurring in groups of several from the same house, and almost all coming from a particular neighborhood.*"

Gerhard decided to follow these cases closely and to examine pathological lesions of those who died of the fever. From nearly 250 cases he was able to conduct about 50 autopsies. In none but one of these were there any lesions like those of typhoid. In fact he was able to conclude - "*in the typhus fever the intestines were more free from lesion than in any other disease accompanied by a febrile movement.*" Patients tended to be residents for some years at Philadelphia, "*their food and mode of living remaining unchanged during that period.*" This added further proof to it not being typhoid, which is "*nearly confined to those persons who had recently removed from one place to another.*" Gerhard was to be stricken by typhoid fever in 1843 at which time he stopped his research to become a practicing physician.

Many physicians in both France and England continued to believe that typhoid and typhus were the same disease. A reviewer of Louis' 1841 edition of his work on typhoid fever, who was aware of Gerhard's work, remained convinced that the continued fevers of both France and England were "*the same species of disease; but that they are different varieties of that species.*" Only when Sir William Jenner demonstrated in London in 1849 the same pathological differences between typhoid and typhus, and furthermore showed that typhus tended to occur in particular households while typhoid did not, and that contracting one form of fever did not protect against the other, was the distinct nature of both diseases well established. He, himself, caught typhus while conducting these studies in 1847 and then typhoid 3 years later.

It would not be until the 1860's that England officially separated typhus from other 'fevers'. In the United States, however, many doctors remained ignorant of typhoid nearly to the end of the century, as reflected by their use of 'typhomalaria' to designate difficult fevers to diagnose.[50]

---

[50] Osler suggested that they could distinguish typhoid from malaria by contrasting the map of Pennsylvania railway with that of the Baltimore-Ohio railway. If the temperature chart ran a relatively smooth course like the former railway then the diagnosis was more

Gerhard knew of the past reputation of typhus when it was known as jail fever, ship fever, camp fever, among other names. He was to witness its contagiousness in his hospital when *"three principle nurses, and about a dozen assistant nurses, besides a number of patients with various diseases were taken with the fever."*[51] In some cases *"the contagion was evidently direct from body to body."* This was believed to have happened when a nurse, who had *"inhaled the breath"* of a patient shortly after having cut his hair, fell ill. This was consistent with Cullen's suggestion that typhus was propagated by human effluvia that had acquired virulence inside the human body.

Gerhard, however, did not believe that typhoid was contagious. Louis had informed him that *"in the course of his long experience of the disease, he had never seen a single case originating in a hospital."* Gerhard had *"seen but one. The contrast between the fevers, in this respect, is obvious."* Gerhard has been faulted for this conclusion, but given Webster's distinction between contagion and infection, he may have been denying typhoid's specific contagiousness, while not denying that under certain circumstances, such as a changing life-style brought about by a changing climate, which he specifically cited as being significant, many people would fall ill around the same time. He may have been ignorant, as well, of the earlier work of Nathan Smith (1762-1829) in which typhoid fever was judged to arise *"from a specific cause, and that cause contagion, and seldom affecting the same person more than once."* More likely, however, he never experienced the disease in a rural context where evidence of its contagious nature was more obvious to see, as exemplified by the experiences of Smith and William Budd (1811-1880).

Smith was attracted to study medicine when at the age of twenty-one years he assisted a surgeon perform an amputation. He apprenticed to that surgeon for the customary three-year period, which qualified him to practice. He then decided to take up medicine and after three years of study at the newly established Harvard Medical School, he received the degree of Bachelor of Medicine. He continued his studies in both Edinburgh and London and returned to establish the medical school at Dartmouth in 1798, with himself in

---

likely to be typhoid, whereas if the chart showed a zigzag course like the latter railway then it was more likely to be malaria!

[51] Bellevue Hospital in New York, during the 1848 outbreak, lost one-third of its assistant physicians from typhus.

charge with only one assistant! Only in 1810 would the Dartmouth trustees appoint a second professor.

Smith published his monograph on typhoid in 1824. He called the disease *typhous fever*. He concluded that typhoid, like smallpox, was contagious, i.e. a disease *"that can be communicated from one individual to another."* He did not collect data systematically nor did he perform any autopsies. Instead, he argued by analogy with smallpox and, most importantly, he rejected the notion of general causes, i.e. those environmental and meteorological causes that Webster had used to demonstrate the infectious (but not contagious) nature of plague, yellow fever and other febrile diseases.

From his own experience Smith knew that certain areas remained disease-free for periods as long as twenty years. If the disease did arise from one or more general, non-specific, factor - *"it is impossible but that some of these circumstances should have occurred"* during this long period of time. Thus typhoid, of which he had found clusters of cases that he had traced to persons who had recently arrived from a community where the disease was already present, had to be caused by a specific agent. Smallpox was known to be contagious but not everyone exposed contracted the disease. So, too, was typhoid able to be transmitted from community to community without everyone falling ill. And both could only be caught once.

Budd's vivid recollections of the typhoid epidemic that struck North Tawton, in July 1839, where he had been born, brought up and was now a practicing physician, left no doubt in his mind, as well, of the contagious nature of this disease. For fifteen years this village of some *"eleven or twelve hundred souls"* had been virtually free of typhoid. Yet this was a village where *"there was no general system of sewers …(and) nothing to separate from the open air the offensive matters which collect around human habitations."* Each cottage or group of cottages had its common privy, *"to which a simple excavation in the ground served as cesspool."* He could testify - *"offensive to the nose, but fever there was none."* For fever to develop, *"a more specific element was needed than either the swine, the dungheaps, or the privies were … able to furnish."* Someone who had fallen sick elsewhere had to introduce that *"specific element"* into North Tawton. Once entrenched, the disease became a *"contagious or self-propagating"* one.

Budd's 1873 publication *Typhoid Fever: Its Nature, Mode of Spreading, and Prevention* provides example after example of similar occurrences. That the disease remained the same in all instances of its study was for him a clear sign of its specificity:

> To propagate itself and no other, and that in a series of indefinite progression, constitutes the very essence of the relation on which the idea of species is founded. How much this implies in the animal and in the plant we all know. It is strange that what it implies in the case of disease should be so seldom recognised.

Specificity implies a specific agent. The specific agents *"are cast off in a material form by the infected body of the fever patient. Some are eliminated from one surface, and some from another."* The morbid product of smallpox is seen in the pustular eruption on the skin; that of phtisis, the tubercle; and that of typhoid, the ulcerations found in the lower end of the small intestine. Typhoid's morbid matter is found in the discharges of the diseased intestine - *"the sewer, which is their common receptacle, is, so to speak, the direct continuation of the diseased intestine."*

Budd only became aware of Bretonneau's paper on typhoid fever in the summer of 1857. There he found, but only in its barest form, the idea that the intestinal affection was *"a true eruption."* However, Budd could not find any evidence that Bretonneau perceived the importance of this fact *"on the mode in which this fever is disseminated."* Convincing evidence of this mode of spread was provided in a number of documented instances in which defective sewerage was shown to have been the cause of a specific outbreak. Nevertheless, when a major outbreak occurred in 1859, in Windsor, the press reported it as an example of *"the true endemic typhoid, not the contagious typhus,"* one caused by *"emanations from the sewers"* of a *"pythogenic"* or *"putrescence"* nature, i.e. from a poison generated by putrescent animal matter. To which Budd reacted:

> To hold ... that the fever which the sewers were communicating was not the effect of the specific fever-poison with which they were so largely supplied, but of some perfectly undefined and purely hypothetical compound which putrefaction is supposed to extricate from the common sewerage, seems to me to be nothing less than to invert all the rules which philosophy and experience have united in showing to be essential to a true induction.

As late as 1873 the contagiousness of typhoid remained a *"great truth"* that was still being disputed. Budd made the pertinent observation that those who opposed its contagious nature had experiences with the disease that was confined to large cities, where *"the operation of contagion ... in not only masked and obscured, but issues in a mode of distribution … which to the superficial observer would appear to exclude the idea of contagion altogether." Also there remained a "continued prevalence of very limited views as to what constitutes evidence of contagion or self-propagation in the case of disease."*

Bretonneau Establishes the Specificity of Diphtheria

Bretonneau believed that each morbid seed caused a special disease, as every seed in natural history gives rise to a determined species, and as every animal or vegetable species has a distinct origin and development, in the same manner every species of disease should receive a specific treatment. (Trousseau on the occasion of Bretonneau's death 1862)

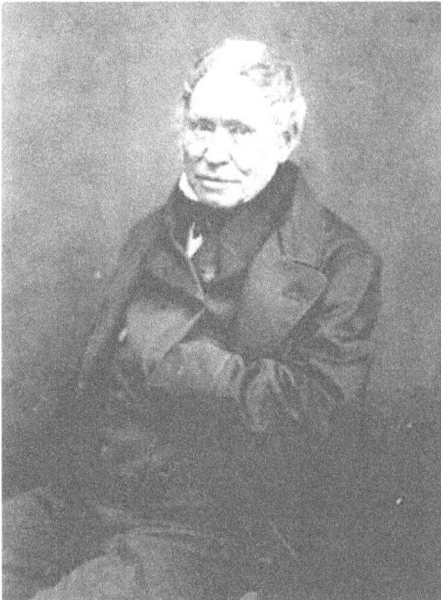

Bretonneau emphasized the specificity of disease more than any of his contemporaries did. The tools he used for his studies were those that had by then become the classic ones of pathological anatomy, i.e. correlating clinical observations with post-mortem findings. But his approach differed from Broussais in that he built his understanding of diphtheria case by case with careful care not to extend his conclusions beyond the evidence that came to light from his examinations and not to be blinded by any pre-conceived ideas.

Bretonneau seemed indifferent to success and was even accused by his students of being lazy. He kept his results to himself and only the pressure of his students pushed him to make them better known. His brilliant pupil, Trousseau, was particularly important in promoting his work.[52] Another student, Alfred Velpeau (1795-1867),

---

[52] For example, it was Trousseau in 1826 who presented Bretonneau's work on typhoid, which he had already begun in 1813. In his presentation Trousseau wished to *"assure Dr. Bretonneau the possession of his discovery, which they have already wished to take from him."*

accused him of being so slow that *"none of your ideas will be yours since others were parceling them out as their own."* As it was, Bretonneau published very little in his lifetime; it was mostly through the diligent efforts of Trousseau and Velpeau that his work became known.

In 1818 an epidemic designated as 'scorbutic gangrene' of the mouth and throat appeared among soldiers in a garrison at Tours. Shortly thereafter, the surrounding civilian population was attacked by 'angina maligna'. It fell on Bretonneau, who was chief physician of the hospital at Tours, to study the epidemic. So fatal was this epidemic that he was able to carry out sixty autopsies in a matter of a few months. The observations that he made and conclusions drawn were published in 1826 in *On Specific Inflammations of Mucous Tissue, and Particularly on Diphtheria, or Membrous Inflammation.*

In the course of his studies, Bretonneau prepared and submitted Memoirs to the Académie Royale de Médecine to which he became a corresponding member in 1824. The first two Memoirs on *Croup and Malignant Angina* were read at the Académie in 1821. In his first Memoir, Bretonneau used a mixture of individual case studies, performed by himself and his assistant, Velpeau, results drawn from dozens of autopsies performed during the epidemic, and the thinking of other physicians who had come to see these diseases as being distinct - to demonstrate that *"scorbutic gangrene of the gums, malignant angina, and croup are only one and the same disease, the phenomena of which present a great diversity of symptoms, according to the functions of the organs affected."*[53]

The second Memoir contains a summary of the specific characters of 'diphtherite' (Bretonneau adopted the term diphtheria at a later time), provides an analysis of historical evidence, and addresses the issue of treatment in which he introduced the effective use of tracheotomy and demonstrated the inefficacy of bloodletting. Of greater relevance is his short section devoted to the question *Is Diphtherite contagious?*

We learn that *"All authors of the 17th century reply to this question in the affirmative."* He cited a dramatic case of a young student in 1625 in Italy who died of the disease after having approached a monk affected with the same

---

[53]Late in the 19th century, it would be shown that scorbutic gangrene of the gums was totally distinct from diphtheria.

malady and acquiescing to the monk's request *"to ascertain if his breath was as fetid as he, himself, believed it to be."*[54]

Turning his attention to the epidemic of Tours, he described how the deaths of twelve children could be linked to the school they all attended, adding this insightful comment:

> *Still it must be admitted that it was often impossible to arrive at the origin of the contagion, and in some circumstances it was altogether improbable that it occasioned the disease. It cannot be denied that the same difficulties might be raised relatively to the transmission of the small-pox, if the contagion of that disease were not established on the most solid foundation. Every time that it has been brought from without into the General Hospital, and that it has propagated itself, it has been easy to ascertain at the beginning, the exact period when it was communicated. But as soon as a certain number of individuals were attacked by it, it became impossible to follow the traces of the contagion through the multitude of indirect and doubtful modes of communication.*

His third Memoir, delivered in November 1825, provided greater clinical details as well as a general account of an epidemic which occurred in 1824 at La Ferrière. Again he called attention to the *"irregularity of the progress of Diphthérite."* He cited a Mr Guersant who wrote that *"the disease sometimes appears suddenly in one of the wards of the Hopital des Enfants, and that it ceases there as soon as three or four have been attacked, but reappears in another ward, after a longer or shorter interruption."* He also quoted from a treatise prepared by Marteau de Grandvilliers, who *"expresses himself on this subject in the most distinct manner:"*

> *This disease, like the smallpox, passes from one village to another, but it does not resemble other epidemics which seize a great number of persons on a sudden, and then pass away like a storm. It attacks in detail, and in this respect it is most treacherous, because it excites less alarm and attracts less attention from those who are appointed to watch over the health of the citizens. In great national maladies, the ministry opens its eyes, and sends assistance; but here the multitude of sick people is not striking, and yet a whole household is insensibly undermined and depopulated. They are the persons who are the most solid hopes of the state, they form the posterity which is to succeed us, who are swept away by this cruel contagion.*

---

[54] Probably the same case discussed in footnote 24.

Bretonneau added again that this *"affection is undoubtedly contagious,"* while asking *"how is the germ which preserves it reproduced?"* a question to which he had no response.

In his fourth Memoir (1826), in which he presents the 1825 epidemic at Chenusson, Bretonneau extended further his concern with the mode by which this disease was transmitted:

> *I have several times received on my face and lips diphtheric concretions discharged to a great distance by the artificial opening of the trachea. I have been struck, in common with a great number of pupils, with the fetid smell exhaled by the breath of some patients. Several attendants at the Hospital had continual communication with them. How did it happen that not one of us was attacked by the disease, when the child who forms the subject of the last case, appears to have contracted it on the occasion of much less intimate association? How was it that the girl Thérèse was alone affected in a ward where there were several other little girls? All these questions have remained as much in doubt as at the period of my first observations.*

The occasion of Bretonneau's fifth Memoir was the pandemic of diphtheria that struck Paris in 1855. He had been asked by his medical colleagues to advise on a form of *"toxaemia which destroy(s) life without closure of the larynx."* He reviewed what he has learned and took the opportunity to expand on the subject of contagion as well as on immunity.

He was distressed to note that the current belief is *"in opposition to truth (and is) repelling any belief in contagions with all the means in its power."* Worse, when contagion becomes too evident to be denied, it is admitted, but with the explanation that *"a disease which was not contagious, may become so under such and such conditions."* To which Bretonneau reacted - *"in the interest of the medical art, it is better that a prominent fact should be forgotten than perverted."*

Bretonneau extended his previous ideas concerning contagion by noting that diphtheria is not carried by air but, instead, by a process analogous to inoculation with smallpox. Those who attend patients cannot contract diphtheria, *"unless the diphtheritic secretion, in the liquid or pulverulent state, is placed in contact with a soft or softened mucous membrane, or with the skin, on a point denuded of epidermis, and this application must be immediate."* He cited the case of a surgeon in his hospital who was inoculated by sputa coughed into his left nostril during an operation. Influenza, being highly prevalent at that time, was thought to have seriously affected the nostrils, predisposing the nasal mucous membranes to the inoculation.

He introduced the notion of immunity by analogy with other poisons (such as opium and tobacco) which if taken bit by bit can be tolerated. Thus, *"physicians who have a large practice, running from one patient to another, and absorbing only fractional portions of virus, succeed in attaining an immunity which is often observed and generally ill-understood."*

Bretonneau's doctrine of specificity was the subject of a lecture given by Trousseau in 1861. In it he impressed upon his readers how wrong Broussais and Brown were in not believing in the specificity of diseases. At the same time he had to acknowledge that while *"we pretend to have shaken the bondage of (their) doctrines, we are still under their influence; our medical ideas, our very language, are deeply affected, despite what we believe."*

Yellow Fever in Europe- To Quarantine or Not?

In my manuscript, the disease of Catalogna will be designated by the name of Typhus amaril, since that of yellow fever has been exclusively reserved for the disease of the Antilles ... although it would be more reasonable to call it Gástrite des inacclimatés. (Rochoux, 1821)

Following Rush's philosophy - to each region its own diseases - Rochoux gave a new name to the outbreak in Catalogna, even though it resembled that of the Antilles. Following Broussais, he designated this new disease as a member of the typhus family (amarillo = yellow in Spanish), and classified it as a gastritis. This particular gastritis was one that struck 'non-acclimated' individuals, i.e. individuals newly visiting areas where 'typhus amaril' was endemic.

During the 18th century yellow fever was largely confined to the coasts of the African and South, Central and North America. It particularly struck down non-immune populations, like the populace of Philadelphia in 1793, where the disease was imported, or the newly arrived French soldiers that tried to suppress the rebellion in Haiti in 1801, where the disease was heavily endemic. France lost as many as 50,000 soldiers, officers, doctors and sailors during the three years that Haiti resisted their attack. The effect of yellow fever on the French was so devastating that it forced Napoleon to abandon whatever thoughts he had of establishing an empire in the Mississippi Valley.

The disease spread along the Atlantic trade routes, brought to new lands by the mosquitoes that bred in the water containers of sailing ships. Of the European countries, Spain was the most heavily affected; it experienced nine epidemics between 1801 and 1821, with an estimated total mortality of 130,000. Both the French and the English became concerned that they had a center of yellow fever right in their 'back yard'.

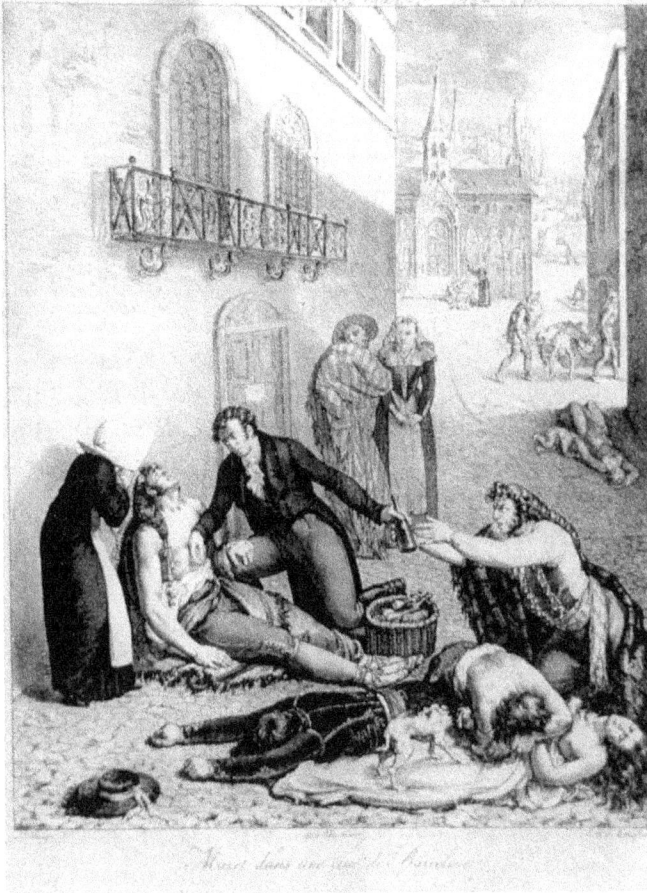

Like Jean Devèze, the French physician who helped run the major yellow fever hospital in Philadelphia during the 1793 epidemic, most French physicians with any experience with the disease were confirmed anti-contagionists. Not only had their own experience in the Caribbean convinced them of the non-contagious nature of yellow fever, they had the support of the anti-contagionist Philadelphia Academy of Medicine that had been

171

founded in 1799. Nevertheless, when a very fatal epidemic of yellow fever broke out in 1821 in Gibraltar, an English 'fortress', the French government and the Academy of Medicine sent a study commission to Barcelona to obtain new information with a view of revising quarantine legislation.

The members chosen by the French government for the commission were all confirmed believers in the contagious nature of yellow fever. They were led by Etienne Pariset (1770-1847), the secretary of the Academy of Medicine. His report dutifully confirmed what the commission was sent to find. For their effort, each member obtained a life pension of 3000 Frs. per year, and a very stringent quarantine law was passed through the chambers in 1822. It was around this time that Nicolas Chervin (1783-1843) returned from America and the Caribbean with his own documented case against contagion. He was recognized as a man of unusual intelligence, one who had made the fight against contagion and quarantines his life work. Even his adversaries spoke highly of him.

Chervin went to Spain to check the accuracy of Pariset's report. He had little trouble documenting how quickly that report had been prepared, thereby forcing the government to reopen the whole question of quarantine. The government passed the question to the Academy of Medicine, which in turn appointed a committee of 18 to examine the issue. After 11 months of deliberation and study, they rejected the position of their secretary and adopted Chervin's point of view; in 1828 he was voted the Grand Prix de Médicine of the Institute.

Chervin documented his position on every occasion that he could. For example, when S. Lassis (1772-1835), shifted from being an anti-contagionist to a contagionist, following the 1821 outbreak, Chervin wrote a short paper on Lassis' *new opinions*. Lassis had come to believe that yellow fever (and plague as well) was everywhere present, but that it only manifested itself as an epidemic when preventive measures were taken against it! Chervin, not too gently, tore his position apart, pointing out, among other things, that Lassis had never left Europe and had never visited any part of the world where plague had ever been present in epidemic form.

In this paper, Chervin very carefully outlined the two opposing positions, those of the contagionists and those of the infectionists, somewhat along the lines that Webster had done 30 years earlier. Contagionists believed that the disease is a product of a germ, or of "*any principle that creates and develops in an individual, and serves afterwards to propagate the sickness among other healthy people, either by contact or by the intermediary of the atmosphere to those nearby."*

Infectionists, including him, believed that yellow fever originates in air *"contaminated by the exhalation of decomposing vegetable and animal matter provoked by high temperature, and probably under a particular meteorological state."* Other unknown causes may be involved. In any case, it can *"never"* be passed on by the sick, even if one approaches or touches them. However, where many people are sick in the same place, they can corrupt the air, but this corruption can only produce typhus and not yellow fever, since yellow fever is due to miasmas created by the chemicals arising from dead matter while the miasmas that cause typhus are the product of living matter.

When a suspected outbreak of yellow fever occurred in Gibraltar in late September 1828, Chervin immediately indicated his availability to go to study it. He even volunteered to go with someone who believed that the disease was contagious arising from a foreign source. Trousseau was chosen to represent the contagionist position. Louis was chosen to represent the Academy of Medicine. The three left France on 1 November of that year, arrived by land on the 20th and started work on the 23rd. They were in a hurry to see cases of the disease since the epidemic was already declining in intensity and could be expected to stop at any moment.

The results of this visit are summarized nicely in a long letter written to a medical colleague by Chervin in June of the following year. In this letter he described in straightforward terms how both the living and autopsy forms of the disease resembled what he had seen in the New World, particularly in the Antilles. All English doctors present with comparable experience shared his views. The next question addressed was whether the disease had been imported or was it of local, indigenous origin. Contagionists argued that it had been imported on the Swedish ship *le Dygden*. Chervin found the notion *"absurd and ridiculous."* What provoked this reaction was the fact that the contagionists had not been able to find any other foreign source for the outbreak in spite of searching hard.

Why seek some remote cause, asked Chervin, when it was obvious that the climatic and environmental conditions of Gibraltar that had prevailed the previous summer had been perfect for breeding a local variant of the disease. The normal summer dry period had lasted from June through September. High humidity and high temperature guaranteed that the vegetable and animal wastes that had accumulated would decompose and give off exhalations that would corrupt the atmosphere. Had any rains fallen, they might have washed the decomposing matter into the sea, but the records showed that this had not been the case. Also, once the exhalations started to rise, they may have been taken away had the winds blown out to the sea, but here too the records showed that prevailing winds were inwards, towards the shore. These winds *"penetrated the sewers and carried the miasmas contained therein directly to the higher part of the town,"* where, not to Chervin's surprise, the first cases of yellow fever had occurred. To this history he added what had been noted during earlier visits, namely, the large number of poor, living under crowded, dirty and unventilated conditions. Better classes were not spared because the whole town had been plunged into a stagnant and immobile atmosphere.

Once yellow fever developed in this manner, could it become contagious? He thought not, since those who came close to the sick were no more affected than any others. Nor did those who did die or fall ill have contact *"with the sick or with so-called contaminated objects."* It was also noted that sporadic cases had occurred earlier, i.e. yellow fever was always present; epidemics would occur if the conditions were right.

And what did Louis and Trousseau have to say? According to Chervin, they had no opinion! They were largely ignorant of the disease. Trousseau had been chosen to participate as a known contagionist. His present *"neutral"* position, Chervin thought was *"already a big change."* Louis, *"as you know, he's a great partisan of ancient medical doctrines that accept the contagiousness of yellow fever as a matter of faith. He's finding it hard to renounce something as fundamental in his beliefs as that,"* but despite trying to prove Chervin wrong, he and Trousseau had failed.

The team stayed until April 15, 1829; Chervin did all he could to have them stay for several weeks more, since he had more studies to conduct. But the others insisted on returning to Paris. One can imagine, after nearly five months of effort, that Chervin's continuing enthusiasm for gathering yet more evidence of the non-contagious nature of yellow fever may have contributed to their determined departure! For Chervin, it would be his last occasion to study yellow fever, since this would be the last large yellow fever outbreak in Europe, with the exceptions of Lisbon in 1857 and Madrid in 1878.

Of additional note in this history is the fact that the 1827 report prepared for the Academy, and favorable to Chervin, was primarily written by Louis René Villermé (1782-1863), the greatest French sanitarian at that time. Villermé had recently published a pioneering and devastating report showing how disease and poverty were strongly correlated in Paris. Later his study of the health conditions of textile workers led in 1841 to the adoption of a law limiting child labor. The localized miasma theory of Chervin suited well Villermé's focus on improving local and working sanitary conditions. This 'collusion' between anti-contagionists and sanitary reformers reached its peak in the middle of the century when the second global wave of cholera reached the New World, as discussed next.

Cholera Reaches the New World

From south to north hath the cholera come,
He came like a despot king;
He hath swept the earth with a conqueror's step,
And the air with a spirit's wing.
We shut him out with a girdle of ships,
And a guarded quarantine;
What ho! now which of your watches slept?
The Cholera's past your line!
There's a curse on the blessed sun and air,
What will he do for breath?
For breath, which was once but a word for life,
Is now but a word for death.
Woe for affection! When love must look
On each face it loves with dread!
The months pass on, and the circle spreads
And the time is drawing nigh
When each street may have a darkened house
Or a coffin passing by.
(ANON. 1832 Canada)

America was fully alert to the imminent arrival of what later would be classified as the world's second cholera pandemic.[55] England's *cordon sanitaire* had been broken in the fall of 1831. The disease soon appeared in various cities of England and Scotland, including London in February 1832. It reached Ireland and Calais, France in March 1832. By 24 March Paris was engulfed in

---

[55] The first pandemic (1817-1823) only reached the borders of Egypt and Russia.

a widespread outbreak; of the first 98 cases, 96 perished. Within 6 months cholera would take more than 18,000 lives there.

The contagious nature of cholera was debated in France, as it soon would be in America. The reality of cholera pushed aside worries about yellow fever. Bretonneau believed cholera to be contagious and protested against the practice of mixing cholera patients with the other cases in the Paris hospitals. Velpeau too voiced his belief in its contagious nature. However, the official position of the Academy of Medicine, reflecting Chervin and the majority of French doctors, was that it was not contagious. Instead, its origin lay in internal infections that were due to miasmas originating under certain climatic and environmental conditions, especially those associated with poor and unsanitary housing.

Throughout the fall and winter of 1831-32, newspapers, magazines and pamphlets kept the American public informed of its deadly progress, as well as the different opinions concerning its cause.[56] When Cholera was announced to have appeared in Quebec and Montreal in June 1832, it was evident that it could only be a matter of days before it would arrive on America's soil. In fact, it had probably arrived earlier but knowledge of its appearance either was unrecognized or suppressed by authorities. By June there was no way of keeping the public ignorant of its presence.

Cholera was particularly rampant in Ireland and of the more than 30,000 emigrants that left Ireland for North America most went to Canada. 50,000 immigrants entered Canada in 1831, and 70,000 to 80,000 were expected in 1832. Quebec received numbers ranging from 600 to 10,000 per week. While there could be little hope that Canada could stem the tide of cholera any better than England had the previous year, fear of cholera forced the Canadian authorities to adapt their 1795 Quarantine Act to this new immediate threat.

The island of Grosse Isle, situated thirty miles below Quebec on the St Lawrence River, was chosen to be the site of the quarantine station where passengers from overseas could be examined and the sick detained in a *lazaretto* (small hospital).[57] Ships that had suffered cholera cases during their

---

[56] There, they learned among other facts, that when cholera reached Austria, people made a pilgrimage to Paracelsus' grave at Salzburg, hoping to be healed by the special powers which, they supposed, were still at his command!

[57] Today this island is a joint Canadian and Irish national monument.

voyage were expected to perform a fifteen-day quarantine, while those arriving with cholera on board were quarantined for thirty days.

The number of incoming ships and immigrants quickly overwhelmed local authorities. Typical numbers of reported deaths due to cholera that occurred at sea during April and May was - *Constantia* - 170 passengers, 29 deaths; *Elizabeth* - 200 passengers, 20 deaths; *Carricks* - 200 passengers, 45 deaths. By the end of June cholera was raging in Quebec. Many cholera-carrying immigrants made their way into America, where it quickly spread along the newly built Erie Canal. Towns and cities in upper New York State, Vermont, and along the Canal invoked quarantine measures, but with no success. Despite the presence of armed militia, immigrants escaped by leaping from halted canal boats, entering the country on foot. New York City knew of its first cases by the end of the same month. Within a matter of weeks more than 2000 deaths were recorded; the total deaths for the epidemic reached 3,500. Before the end of the year, cholera was to reach all parts of the country connected by rail, canals, sail and steamboats.

This was cholera's first visitation to the New World; local authorities recent decades of experience with yellow fever provided little guidance to build on for their imminent battle with this new pestilential disease. However, New York's temporary committees of the 1790's had evolved by then into a permanent Board of Health that consisted of the Board of Alderman meeting with the mayor and recorder. Its first response was the establishment of a committee to gather information from Europe and Canada. Quarantine against most of Europe and Asia was proclaimed in early June. No ship could approach closer than three hundred yards to the city and no vehicle closer than a mile and a half without the permission of the Board of Health. On June 13th New York's sanitation system was overhauled to allow the city to better enforce the cleaning of its streets.

In July the Board established a Special Medical Council which was manned by seven of the city's more prominent physicians. The City's first of five cholera hospitals was ready to receive the sick in July as well, but only weeks after the first recognized cases of cholera had appeared. Various other preventive measures were debated and acted upon to the degree that local politics and commerce allowed. Medical advisors urged that hydrants be run several times a week during the summer to help keep the streets clean. Streets, private sinks, yards, and cesspools should be disinfected with chloride and lime or quicklime. The sale of fruit should be stopped as well as all saloons closed.

The city's worst slums were evacuated and temporary shanties erected in a half-dozen places to house the displaced poor. During the summer of 1832 New York became cleaner than it had been at any time in the memory of its inhabitants. Nevertheless, not all streets were cleaned and the dead piled up and overwhelmed the city's capacity to bury them quickly. Fortunately, the disease waned quickly and by August 28 New York was pronounced *"safe."*

In the short time of its existence, the 1832 epidemic of cholera provoked the same debate of earlier yellow fever epidemics - was it a contagious disease? was a quarantine called for? how could one protect oneself?

There was no doubt as to how terrible a disease cholera was; it sometimes proved fatal within hours following its first symptoms. Its link with filth and poverty was demonstrated again and again. It was a 'poor man's plague', striking everywhere the most destitute and weak. Almost all who died in New York that summer were buried at the Potter's Field or in St. Patrick's cemetery. Overlaid with its association with poverty, cholera was also seen to be a disease of an immoral, sinful life. Prostitutes were singled out as being its most ready victims. Those who indulged in drink, gluttony and sexual excess risked their lives, a risk that many saw as a divine imposition.

Many doctors did not recognize cholera as a new disease. Some saw it as a variant to already familiar ailments. Daniel Drake (1785-1852), one of the most observant of all America's 19th century physicians, claimed that cholera bore to "cholera morbus" (a flexible term that covered most dysenteries and diarrheas), a relation similar to that of influenza to a common cold."[58] Such associations argued for familiar treatment - bloodletting, calomel, laudanum, sometimes singly, often together. More radical treatments included tobacco smoke enemas, electric shocks and the injection of saline solutions into the veins. The injection of saline solutions was new and considered by some to be one of the most rational and successful modern treatments of cholera.[59]

---

[58] This did not prevent him from being the only member of an eight member sanitary commission to announce at the onset of an epidemic that in 1832 would end up killing 571 people in the Cincinnati population of 30,000 that it was *"epidemic cholera,"* and not *"the usual exciting causes of bowel affections."*

[59] Today oral rehydration therapy is an essential feature in the prevention of deaths during a cholera epidemic. It took more than a century for scientists to work out the correct route

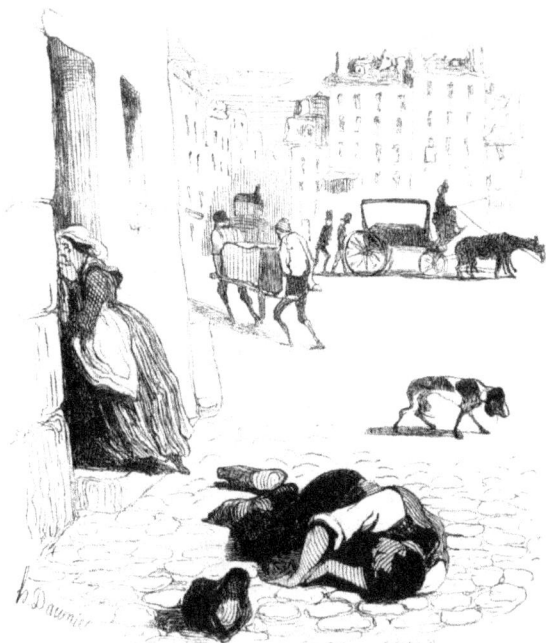

Ah! sans l'heureux secours des mille démentis !

Contre tous les Jonnès de tous côtés partis,

Une heure de soupçon, de doute ou de silence

19th Century

The miasmatic school of cholera's origin led to the abandonment of centrally located graveyards. Deemed too unhealthy, owing to the air of decomposition that arose from them, American cemeteries began to be situated outside town limits in the early 1830s.[60]

Although quarantine was established, many physicians insisted that cholera was not contagious. This position followed that of Anglo-Indian physicians who reported on the 1817 epidemic in India and the vast majority of European doctors. As was the case with yellow fever, the general public thought otherwise. If they could afford to do so, people fled their communities with the first appearance of cholera. Of New York's 220,000 population, more than 70,000 were estimated to have left the city during the summer of 1832. In fleeing they took cholera with them to the interior; some 800 more were judged to have died while away from the City.

Philadelphia's long history with yellow fever led that city to be almost indifferent to the approach of cholera. Her medical faculty, having so thoroughly convinced itself of the local or 'malarious' development of the disease, concentrated on purifying the city. No *cordons sanitaires* were put in place around the city nor were any restrictions placed on travel between that

---

for replacing lost body salts and liquids, as well as the correct mix of sugar and salt to ensure their rapid and effective absorption.

[60] As early as the 16th century the Paris Faculty of Medicine on several occasions urged the closure of the great Cemetery of the Innocents, situated well within the city walls, as a sanitary measure.

city and New York. Philadelphia suffered much less than New York; less than 900 deaths were recorded, almost all among the poor. Had they avoided eating watermelons and green corn, the number of dead would have been less, or so local physicians claimed.

(CINCINNATI CHRONICLE-EXTRA)

CURE OF CHOLERA.

Fellow Citizens,

Would you be cured of Cholera take the disease in time.

It begins with some sort of Bowel Complaint or disturbance of the stomach. In this stage it is easily cured; and all who neglect this stage are in danger of perishing.

Whoever has a lax or sickness at stomach, or Colic, should instantly take to his bed, in a warm room and drink hot tea of sage, balm, or Thorough wort, or even hot water-bathing his feet if cold, and applying a warm poultice over the bowels.

Without this nothing will do any good-All who go about in the damp air after the bowel complaint has set in will get Cramps and Spasms and die--I again say they will die!

Besides what I have mentioned, they should take a powder, of ten grains of Calomel and one of Opium mixed, if grown persons, and children should take less in proportion; or a teaspoonful of powdered Rhubarb.

They should, also, take a tea-spoonful, every hour, of the Aromatic Camphorated water, which Is a cheap article, and may be had of most of the Apothecaries.

All who are of a full habit, or have Fever, or Colic should be bled.

Again let me warn every one, that the dreadful Epidemic commences as a mild bowel complaint, and in that stage may be cured-when vomiting coldness and spasms com-bined, come on, death will follow-has followed, in almost every case that has yet occurred in the city. He who goes about with a mild complaint upon him should expect to perish.

The Epidemic would loose all its terrors, if people would attend, instantly, to the first symptoms-Go to bed, drink hot water or tea, promote a perspiration, and send for their family Physician.

Terror is a great exciting cause. The disease prod uced by terror requires treatment. Let no one presume to laugh another out of his fears. All the terrified should take to their beds-this will best counteract its bad effects.

Let all who read what is here written, recount it to their friends. Let us unite in aiding each other, for a few days--the Pestilential Cloud will soon pass away. The disease, absolutely, is not catching.

Daniel Drake. M. D.

Cincinnati, Saturday afternoon October 13th-1832

A reconstructed facsimile of the original in the Transylvania Library

When a contingent of doctors from Philadelphia visited Canada in June to study the epidemic, they returned even more convinced of the local, miasmatic nature of cholera. The pestilence was clearly caused, in their eyes, by a poison in the air - effluvia, miasmas, mal-aria - which arose from the 'bowels of the earth', from decaying animal or vegetable matter or from the bodies of the unclean or the sick. An experiment conducted at Montreal demonstrated the presence of such effluvia. A piece of fresh beef, hung upon the highest steeple in the city, was said to have become putrid in thirty minutes. The atmosphere, having thus been made miasmatic, would make ill those weakened with worry, or 'excited' from having eaten one of the forbidden fruits or from exposure to cold, dampness, or the night air.

* * * * *

The influenza pandemics of the previous century had given rise to numerous exotic theories to explain its movement and distribution. By now, the reader will no longer be surprised to learn that comparable theories emerged following cholera's second global appearance in Europe and the America's. My favorite image is found in Wood's write-up on epidemic cholera where he attempts to explain how it is that two ships had left Europe with all crew members and passengers healthy only to be attacked with cholera while at sea:

> *The two vessels, departing from a healthy port in Europe, entered at a certain period of their passage the cholera atmosphere, which, in the regular progress of the epidemic, was making its way westward over the Atlantic. With this atmosphere, impregnated with the germs of the cholera cause, the whole capacity of the two vessels was totally imbued. They outsailed the advancing column of aerial poison, and carried the germs of it with them to the places of their destination. At Staten Island, these germs propagated in the air; but the reproduction soon ceased, either through the influence of cold, or from the want of a due medium for the process. At New Orleans, on the contrary, finding favouring influences in the hot weather, and probably in the state of the atmosphere, the cause multiplied with vast rapidity, and, being carried by the steamboats up the river, diffuse itself in the towns which stud the banks of that river and its tributaries.*

Only in the following spring (1849) did the "*regular course of its progress (get re-established)…The column of morbific influence through which the ships had passed, and which thy had outsailed, had now reached our continent.*"

The ability of individuals to carry the disease with them on their clothing was accepted by Wood, but only "*in some rare instances*" would this route lead to a spread of the disease. *"But this is not contagion (since) the effect would ensue as well from a healthy as from a diseased person."*[61]

Wood's description of the 'cholera atmosphere' is taken from his 1858 textbook. In 1859, the English physician, John Parkin, Late Medical Inspector for Cholera in the West Indies, opposed this theory on the following grounds:

> *How, we may ask, was this ...poison-cloud ... transported from the East to the West? By the winds? Assuredly not; for this disease has progressed as regularly against, as with the wind. Across the continent of India it traveled at the rate of a degree a-month - its progress being the same against as with the strong and violent monsoon...Now, if a poison-cloud had been in the air of these localities, would it not, we may ask, have been dispersed, in the same number of months, to the four quarters of the globe? Such assuredly would have been the case; and we may therefore conclude that this winged messenger of death has no existence, excepting in the fertile imagination of those who required a pivot on which to hang their otherwise defenseless theory.*

Parkin favored a theory that some *"disturbance in the physical world,"* e.g. volcanic action, had instigated *"a new period in the medical history of the world - an epidemic period - characterised ... by disease and pestilence in the animal and vegetable creation..."* This same 'epidemic period' was responsible for other epidemic outbreaks as well, helping to explain, for example, the appearance in the West Indies of remittent fever *"among the black population, a class of persons who, under ordinary circumstances, are exempt from fever."* The resemblance of his theory with that of Webster is striking.

Specific Modes of Transmission for Cholera and Yellow Fever Lost in the 'Sanitary Idea' and Conflicting Causation Theories

> *As cholera commences with an affection of the alimentary canal ... it follows that the morbid material producing cholera must be introduced into the alimentary canal - must, in fact, be swallowed accidentally...(Snow)*

> *All smell is disease. (Chadwick)*[62]

---

[61] It would not be until the 1890s that healthy disease carriers would be demonstrated for cholera and other diseases. This critical finding helped explain many outbreaks that 'jumped' from one community to another without touching those in between (as also occurs in outbreaks of diphtheria, for example).

The cholera germ-bearing excrements which penetrate into porous and otherwise suitable layers of the soil, by the fine subdivision which they experience modify the existing processes of decay and decomposition in the soil in such a way that in addition to the normal gases of putrefaction a specific Cholera-Miasm is developed, which is then spread along with other exhalations into the houses. (Pettenkofer)

Pettenkofer's theory is couched ... in terms so vague and mysterious that I never myself feel quite sure of exactly understanding what it involves. (Budd)

John Snow (1813-1858) did for cholera what Budd had done for typhoid, namely demonstrate that ingesting contaminated water caused the disease. He started studying cholera during 1831 when it first invaded England. At that time he was an 18-year-old apprentice to a country physician who served several mining towns. Snow noted that the miners, who frequently were stricken by cholera, lacked access to sanitary latrines and washing facilities. In 1849 he could affirm that 'bad air' did not carry the disease since the intestines were affected not the lungs. Instead, he argued, it was carried in the excreta and vomits of cholera patients on unwashed hands and shared food:

The bed linen nearly always becomes wetted by the cholera evacuations and the hands of persons waiting on the patient become soiled without them knowing it; they must accidentally swallow some of the excretion, and leave some on the food they handle or prepare, which has to be eaten by the rest of the family, who, amongst the working class, often have to take their meals in the sickroom...

---

[62] The association of bad odors with disease is probably as old as any of the ideas discussed. Odors occupy an important place in the theories of all Neo-Platonic and Hermetic philosophers. By the 19th century, however, this association probably had lost any 'philosophical' meaning.

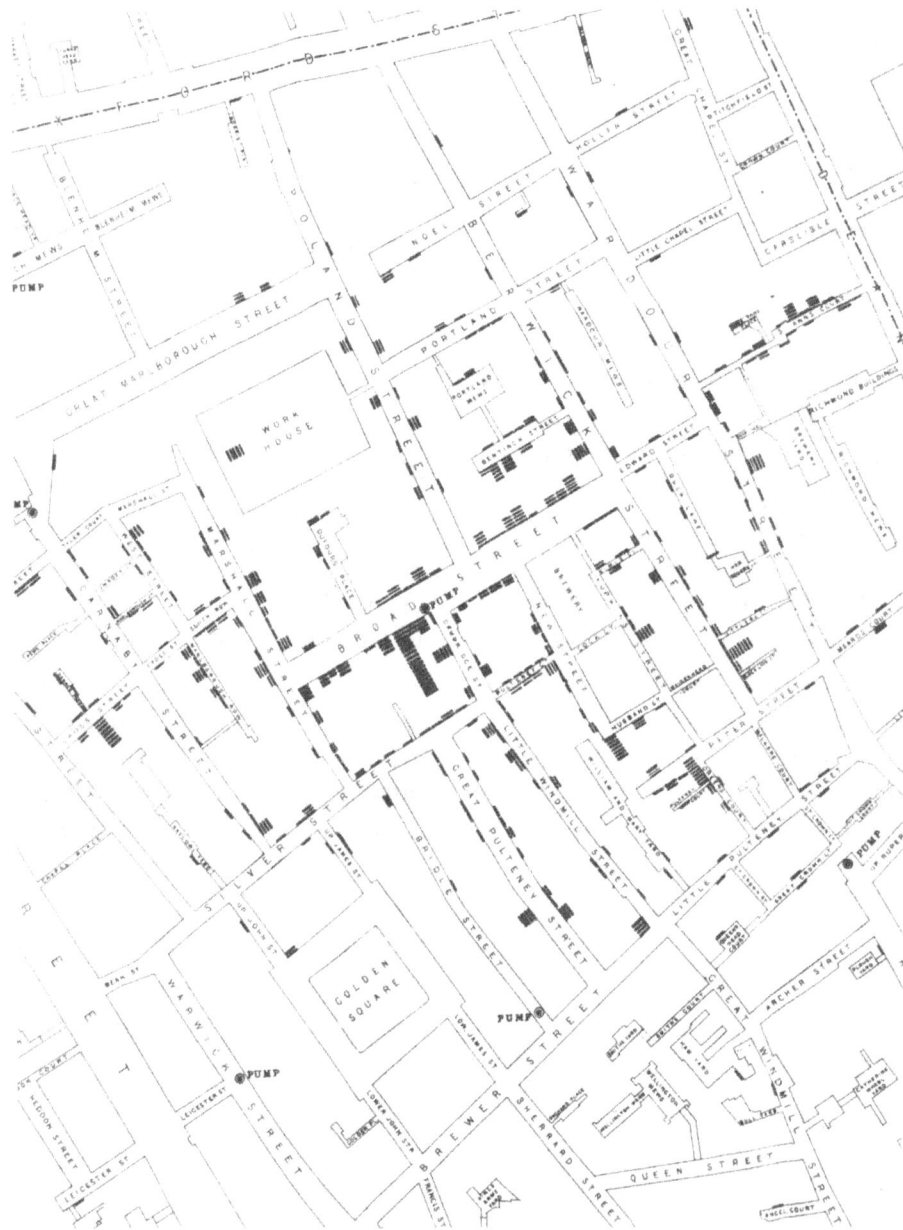

But cholera was not only confined to the poor, it also reached the well-to-do members of the community. For this to happen Snow alluded to *"the mixture of the cholera evacuations with the water used for drinking and culinary purposes,*

either by permeating the ground, and getting into wells, or by running along channels and sewers into the rivers from which entire towns are sometimes supplied with water."

The 1854 cholera epidemic, which Snow described as *"the most terrible outbreak of cholera which ever occurred in this kingdom,"* provided him the chance to confirm his speculations. By careful study of a particularly fatal outbreak confined within a radius of 250 yards he was able to link deaths to one source of water - a street pump on Broad Street supplying the affected area. He persuaded the local Board of Guardians to remove the handle of that pump and the epidemic shortly ceased.

More convincing, since the epidemic was already waning when the pump was disabled, was his case by case investigation of each death. He found a gentleman who had visited his brother for only twenty minutes (drinking the local water) before returning to Brighton where he was attacked the next evening. Particularly striking was the fact that a Mrs Eley died from cholera, along with her niece who had visited her earlier, despite the fact that neither had visited the district in months, but having a special fondness for the Broad Street water, she had her son deliver a bottle of it daily. There were no other cases of the disease in either of the communities where these women lived.

Snow's first cholera investigations appeared in his *On the Mode of Communication of Cholera* published in 1849. Later results and explanations were published in 1855, at which time he had become a prominent physician and London's leading anesthetist. He died shortly thereafter. Budd's first paper on typhoid fever was a short paper published in 1857, followed by a series of papers. His definitive book on the subject was published in 1873. Although both attracted attention and no doubt followers, their findings had little impact on the sanitary reform that was then in place. Snow died at the early age of 45 and thus had little time to use his strong position to promote his ideas. Budd was a provincial practitioner, so his views aroused little interest and had no impact on how the spread of both cholera and typhoid were understood. In any case, their views were lost in the 'sanitary idea' of Edwin Chadwick (1800-90), mastermind of the sanitary movement that had emerged earlier under his leadership in the 1830s.

Chadwick was a lawyer who was a student and disciple of Jeremy Bentham (1748-1832), the father of the New Poor Law enacted in 1834, and philosopher of Utilitarianism - the use of social policy to bring about the 'greatest happiness of the greatest number'. Chadwick is said to have inherited his mentor's energy and zeal as well as arrogance and abrasiveness, making him a rather forceful and dominating personality. Early in the course of his efforts to improve the productivity of England's poorer working class he came to believe that much poverty was due to disease and thus the success of the new law would depend on improving the health of the poor. In 1837 he turned his attention to public health.

With the help of three doctors sympathetic to sanitary reform Chadwick gathered evidence for the *Report on the Sanitary Condition of the Labouring Population of Great Britain* which was published in 1842. The conditions that he described were those of an *"unknown country,"* facts that the *"persons of the wealthier classes"* did not or would not know about - foul odors of open cesspools; garbage, excrement, and dead rats rotting in the streets; filth and scum floating on the river; and sewage passing as drinking water. Chadwick's principle concern was the 'miasma' emanating from all that decaying matter, the 'fetid effluvia', 'poisonous exhalations', and 'reeking atmosphere' that undermined the physical, moral and mental well being of the poor.

In 1838 Chadwick secured a new law requiring the registration of causes of death and selected William Farr (1807-83) to administer its operation. Farr brought to his work the same enthusiasm and dedication possessed by Chadwick. Although he had studied medical statistics under Louis in Paris, where he would have concentrated on correlating autopsy findings with diagnostic and therapeutic ones, he joined his colleagues in assigning greater importance to environmental determinants to health, particularly crowding. His statistics provided the ammunition that Chadwick needed to pursue his reforms. A new Royal Commission on the Health of the Towns was established in 1843. In 1848, under the threat of the advancing second global wave of cholera, the newly passed Public Health Bill received royal consent in August. One week later the first case of cholera was announced.

In 1852 Farr published his *Report on the Mortality of Cholera in England, 1848-9*. Its 100-page introduction is followed by 400 pages of tables, maps and diagrams. Nine 'cholera fields' were identified, each one centering on a large port city. More than 80% of the registered 53,000 deaths in 1849 occurred among 40% of the population who lived on 14% of the land. Concerning environmental factors, his statistics showed that the mortality of cholera varied inversely with elevation. He, still thinking in miasmatic terms, concluded that this could be explained by the higher atmospheric pressure present at sea level.[63] Surprisingly, however, cholera mortality did not seem to vary directly with population density as general mortality had some years earlier.

While Farr was preparing his 1852 report, Max von Pettenkofer (1818-1901), one of the greatest sanitarians of the last century, began to take an interest in cholera.[64] Before his long career ended he would write more than 1000 pages about cholera. He incorporated typhoid fever as well in the theories that he developed, relying mostly on results obtained by other investigators.

The fact that cholera spread along well-traveled lines of communication led him to accept that a contagious factor was involved in its spread. Like Snow, he accepted that this factor was human excretal discharges, but unlike him, he did not believe that water was the medium through which contagion operated. He had ruled out the atmosphere since cholera cases often fail to produce other cases in the immediate community and it often spread against prevailing winds. Instead he insisted that the dissemination of the disease took place only in the presence of 'suitable' soil.[65] All of his research aimed to gather evidence in support of this hypothesis.

Pettenkofer demonstrated that a canary could survive between two layers of soil. This along with other studies showed how air permeates the soil, and thus how the cholera poison that he believed arose from fermentation in the soil could reach human communities. Only soil suitably humid could act to develop such cholera-carrying miasma:

Cholera is produced by the development of a gas through the decomposition of liquid excremental discharges (arising from either urine or feces) in moist, porous layers of the soil (or some equivalent material). The discharge

---

[63] Farr grouped diseases that he believed were essentially due to filth and poverty. He called them 'zymotic' diseases, reflecting Liebig's concept of disease as analogous to fermentation (discussed later). Only under the right circumstances would the disease-causing fermenting matter be released into the atmosphere.

[64] He is noted, among other accomplishments, for his development of the first large city pure-water system, in Munich Germany.

[65] Hirsch's 1882 write-up on Asiatic cholera provides extensive evidence gathered by many investigators in support of Pettenkofer's views. Snow's work, while looked on sympathetically, is covered briefly and is said to be lacking proof owing to the possibility that *"drinking water may have been fouled with excrementitious matters, especially the alvine dejecta…"*

> *in question must come from human beings who have suffered in greater or less degree from symptoms of cholera or perhaps from those who have merely come from places where cholera is epidemic.*

Much of his studies showed that high-lying communities residing on solid bed-rock rarely were attacked by cholera while low-lying communities with extensive natural drainage were often prone to cholera epidemics. He incorporated Farr's 1848-49 data to support his ideas. He concluded that ideal conditions were ones where the soil alternated between dry and moist states. Also taken, as a confirmation of his theory, was the observation that ozone disappeared from the air during a cholera epidemic.

Pettenkofer argued strongly against any general system of quarantine or any specific efforts to isolate those sick with cholera or efforts to disinfect excreta. Instead, he advocated sanitation - sewerage and water-supply - "*These two well-proven methods so operate that the soil of a city is much less polluted by the discharges of human households and that the variation in the moisture content of the soil layers is greatly reduced.*"

Pettenkofer's conclusion that efforts to disinfect excreta were useless contrasts in the extreme with that of Budd. Budd understood well that Pettenkofer was claiming that the poison of fever was not "*like the poison of small-pox and the other contagious fevers, cast forth from the body in a finished state...*" and that fermentation, which did not communicate "*any new property to the essential agent ... probably has the principal hand in hastening the extrication and liberation of the germs in which the infective power resides.*" Budd, himself, did allow for the possibility that a poison cast upon the ground could find its way into humans "*by emanations borne upon the air.*" But none of this, in his eyes, diminished one bit the value of disinfection - "*the one great means whereby the spread of typhoid fever may be prevented.*"

So firmly a believer was Pettenkofer in his ideas that he was not disturbed at all when Robert Koch (1843-1910) discovered the cholera vibrio bacillus in 1883. From his earliest conception of the disease, he had postulated the presence of some 'matter' that was implicated in the subsequent spread of the disease. In 1869, 14 years before Koch isolated the cholera vibrio, he had conjectured that cholera, as well as typhoid fever, involved specific microorganisms. But, according to his theory, more than just the organism was needed to cause disease. To 'prove' this, on 7 October 1892 he drank a fresh culture of cholera vibrio that had been isolated from a dying patient. No symptoms developed other than a "*light diarrhea with an enormous proliferation of the bacilli in the stool."* He thanked Koch for having provided him with the *"so-called cholera vibrio,"* while informing him that he remained *"in his usual good health."*

His having had cholera in 1830 is thought to have provided him some degree of immunity. A different explanation for the lightness of his attack is that Koch, anticipating Pettenkofer's self-experiment, had managed to dilute the culture before passing it on! However, others repeated the experiment, including Rudolph Emmerich and Elie Metchnikoff, with more serious, but not fatal, consequences. Emmerich would succeed Pettenkofer at the University of Munich; Metchnikoff would later win a Nobel Prize for his studies on immunology.[66]

An intriguing aspect of Pettenkofer's mistaken views concerning cholera was his early (1855) and correct conjecture that healthy individuals could be carriers of the disease. He used the possibility that a healthy individual could carry and then transmit cholera to counter Snow's 'proof' that the Broad Street pump was responsible for the local outbreak of cholera. By telling of similar instances where visitors had brought the disease with them, he concluded - *"Mrs. Eley might have been infected through the intercommunication of her son ... without the intervention of drinking water."* (emphasis added) It does not seem that Pettenkofer used the revolutionary notion of the healthy carrier to argue against quarantine, an argument that might have offered a different meeting ground for both proponents and opponents of contagion and quarantine.

Pettenkofer committed suicide in 1901 following a period of sickness and depression. Although nearly 20 years had passed from Koch's discovery of the cholera vibrio, there still remained strong support for his theories so it is doubtful that his decision to take his life was related to his having been wrong concerning cholera and typhoid. Yet he was wrong and that mistake caused some major public health errors where his followers did not keep water supply systems as clean as they should have, as witness the typhoid epidemic of 1901 in Germany and the cholera epidemic of 1911 in Naples, Italy.

---

[66] Pettenkofer was far from being the first doctor to attempt through 'self-experimentation' to dramatically demonstrate that certain diseases were not contagious. Almost a hundred years earlier Desgenettes had auto-innoculated himself with plague; numerous yellow fever self-experiments took place as well as others with plague and cholera. Amazingly almost all of these proved not to be fatal.

Plague Legends

In late 1901 there was a typhoid epidemic in Gelsenkirchen, a town in the Ruhr valley of Germany. More than 3000 people fell ill, of whom 8% died. The outbreak became a subject of an official investigation during which both Koch and Emmerich were called to testify. Koch and other expert witnesses maintained that the outbreak was due to the mixing of impure Ruhr water into the city's water system. Emmerich repudiated this idea. Remaining totally faithful to his predecessor, he testified - *"Gentlemen, it is my firm, solemn conviction that water plays no role here, but that soil-relationships carry responsibility."*

The trial had become possible under a German law of 1879 that made it a penal offence to purvey foodstuffs that could be injurious to health. The first line of the defense was that water was not a foodstuff. Koch argued to the contrary and was upheld by the judge. The defense then tried unsuccessfully to impugn Koch's credibility! Then matters hinged on the validity of Pettenkofer's theories. Finally the defense argued that the epidemic was an Act of God and that Pettenkofer's theory, which they claimed was still valid, was not something that a jury could decide. After weeks of testimony, the Water Company was fined for having adulterated the water supply. No statement was made concerning validity of either Pettenkofer's or Koch's theories.

Naples suffered a major outbreak of cholera in 1884 when more than 14,000 people died. So great was the social and economic impact that the government decided to invest heavily in a plan to clear the slums and improve the sewerage and water systems. Believing in Pettenkofer's theory that contaminated soil was necessary for the cholera germ to be converted into a disease-carrying miasma, the plan called primarily for the removal of the sewage from the subsoil to stop the miasma from being produced. Providing pure water was secondary. The system that was put in place was inadequate and the next pandemic wave of cholera that hit Europe in 1911 evoked yet another major outbreak in this city. This was not the last remnant of Pettenkofer's errors. Even as late as 1917 there were books concerning public health which still gave credence to his cholera and typhoid fever etiology theories.

It is perhaps fitting to end this history with the fact that the fifth cholera pandemic, which provided Koch in 1883 the opportunity to demonstrate that the disease was caused by a comma-shaped organism, gave rise in 1892 to a large outbreak in Hamburg that offered rather conclusive evidence of how wrong Pettenkofer's ideas were. Hamburg, a self-governing city within the new German Reich, drew its water from the Elbe without special treatment. Immediately adjacent to Hamburg lay the Prussian town of Altona, where a water-filtration plant was in operation. When cholera broke out in Hamburg, Altona was totally spared. The soil of both towns was as close as any earth could be, and both shared identical air. Only a matter of water filtration separated the one from the other.

Apparent Water, Soil and Air Sources of the Malarial Fever

All other circumstances being equal, autumnal fever prevails most where the amount of organic matter is greatest, and least where it is least... decaying matter is one of the conditions necessary to the production of autumnal fever. As to the mode in which it cooperates, two opinions may be entertained: First. It may supply the material out of which a poisonous gas is formed; and, Second, It may be a nidus or hot-bed of animalcules or vegetable germs. (Drake)

Hippocrates did not have a 'global view' when he formulated his miasmatic theory. Nor did he have yellow fever and cholera to contend with. Even the presence of plague is not certain as noted earlier. To the disease specialists in the 19th century, who had these and other epidemic diseases to contend with, malaria was clearly different. It did not seem to move from one country to another. Thus the morbific atmosphere that caused other diseases to be present did not seem to generate malaria. Even when carried by the winds, its spread was confined to a distance of several miles, at most. In short, it was the most local miasmatic disease of them all.

As reflected in the above quote, taken from Drake's *A Systematic Treatise, Historical, Etiological, and Practical, on the Principal Diseases of the Interior Valley of North America, as They appear in the Caucasian, African, Indian, and Esquimaux Varieties of Its Population*, by the mid 19th century malaria's miasma was understood to be either a poisonous gas, a vegetable germ or an animalcule. Drake's most remarkable manuscript was published in two volumes in 1850 and 1854, totaling 1863 pages. Malaria, or the autumnal fever, as Drake preferred to call it, occupied the most important place.

Drake was by all accounts an exceptional individual. Born in humble circumstances in New Jersey, he grew up in poverty in the wilderness of Kentucky, and started his studies at the age of 15 in Cincinnati, where he was its first medical student. He received a diploma four years later that qualified him to practice medicine and he became a partner with his mentor, Dr William Goforth. Although Goforth was a follower of John Brown's theories, Drake tended towards those of Rush, whom he heard lecture in the medical department of the University of Pennsylvania. In 1815 he returned to Philadelphia for further study and to obtain his medical degree. Later in his career he would turn against Rush's violent therapy and became a champion of moderate dosage.[67]

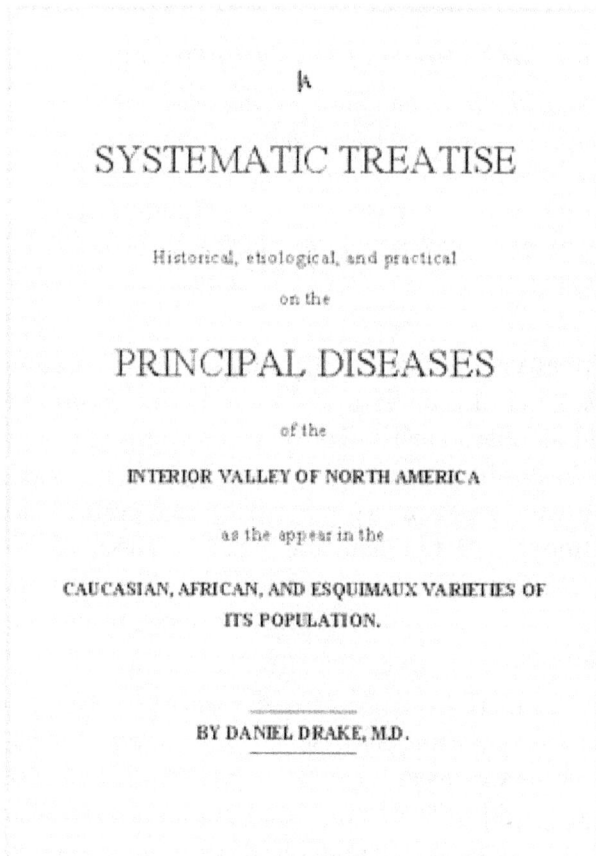

A

SYSTEMATIC TREATISE

Historical, etiological, and practical

on the

PRINCIPAL DISEASES

of the

INTERIOR VALLEY OF NORTH AMERICA

as the appear in the

CAUCASIAN, AFRICAN, AND ESQUIMAUX VARIETIES OF ITS POPULATION.

BY DANIEL DRAKE, M.D.

Drake had a long teaching career and was deeply involved in all sorts of civic activities in Cincinnati. There he helped found a library, a debating club, and a natural museum, for which he hired an unknown naturalist, John James Audubon, as one of its curators. Like Rush, he attacked slavery, and the excessive use of alcohol. These activities brought him wealth and local prominence. His relationship with his medical colleagues, however, was turbulent, to say the least. His quick temper and brusque way was not popular; he was challenged to a duel on several

---

[67] One advantage Drake had over Rush, which may have reduced his reliance on 'heroic' measures, was the fact that quinine, the most active ingredient of Peruvian bark, had been isolated by two French scientists in 1820 and was available in standard amounts. Treatment with 120g of bark, which often provoked vomiting and subsequent failure, was equivalent to about 2g of quinine tablets.

occasions, which he declined.

From an early age Drake was attracted to the study of nature. His interest in the epidemiology of disease seems to have been prompted by an epidemic of what was probably typhoid fever around 1806. From that time he constantly studied the relationship of climate, geography and botany to disease. Before he developed his own views on the origin of diseases, he advised physicians to rely on Webster's *"learned, but neglected work on epidemic diseases."*

In 1808 Drake wrote a short account of the typhoid fever epidemic in Kentucky. He followed this in 1810 with a longer piece on the diseases of Cincinnati, in which he described its topography, geology, climate and condition. This was so successful that he published a greatly expanded version in 1816. Other publications followed, which included not only those related to diseases but ones that focussed on the history and character of the people in America's West. He identified with the West and its frontier. Out of this identification came the idea to take as his subject the whole central plain of America, the thousands of square miles between Lake Superior and the Gulf of Mexico, and between the Allegheny and the Rocky Mountains. Over a ten year period, starting around 1840, he studied its topography, meteorology, oceanography, geology, anthropology, history, political institutions, botany, and of course its diseases. During this period he travelled over 30,000 miles, visiting *"the cities and towns of the Middle West, the villages and hamlets of the basin of the Mississippi, the settlements of the colonist, the reservations and wigwams of the Indian, the campfires of the trappers, the barracks of the frontier posts, the mines of the unexplored West."* It is from these visits that he wrote his *'Systematic Treatise'*, referred to above.

Everywhere in the 'Interior Valley' of America, he found the fevers of malaria, known under different names - *"autumnal, bilious, intermittent, remittent, congestive, miasmatic, malarial, marsh, malignant, chill-fever, ague, fever and ague, dumb ague, and, lastly the Fever."* He reduced the cause of malaria to three possibilities. Either it was a poison that took the form of an inorganic gas or a germ of animalculus or vegetable nature (the two hypotheses reflected in the opening quote of this section), or it was the *"direct, combined action of a hot, humid, and electrical atmosphere."* He related the first two to soil conditions, while the third, which he termed the *"meteoric (weather) hypothesis"*, involved the *"direct, combined action of a hot, humid and electrical atmosphere."* The advocates of the latter hypothesis *"deny the existence of a special poison."* He examined each of the three hypotheses drawing upon observations he and others had made concerning where malaria was and was not to be found.

Drake quickly dispensed with the 'meteoric' hypothesis, arguing that malaria must have a cause, one which *"must be a poison, dissolved or suspended in (the atmosphere)."* He cited twelve situations that argue against *"some conjunction of the ordinary elements and sensible qualities of the atmosphere"* being malaria's cause. Autumnal fever seldom appears on board of vessels whose air is saturated with vapor. Inhabitants of malarious areas breathe a similar atmosphere of nearby areas that are much less afflicted with the Fever. In many parts of Kentucky and Tennessee, where the surface is dry and ridgy and the streams narrow or tortuous, the Fever occurs although the atmospheric humidity is small. Single families settling in forests are free from malaria but when several families arrive and *"an extensive breaking up of the soil takes place,"* malaria begins to prevail, *"although the heat and moisture are not thereby increased."* Persons who have lodged only for a single night in certain localities have been taken down by the Fever some time afterwards. Some have been seized in the spring with intermittents living where there is no malaria. These *"remote"* effects are *"in no degree characteristic of heat and moisture."*

Drake's belief in the importance of soil conditions is in evidence throughout his travels. His visit to Memphis, Tennessee, for example, led him to observe that the *"cretaceous bluffs on one side of the Mississippi, and the low alluvial bottom on the other, afford to its physicians many opportunities for studying the comparative characters, prevalence, and type of autumnal fevers on the two kinds of surface."* Also, he found the Green River basin, in Kentucky, comparatively free of swamps but prone to autumnal fever due to *"the pools formed in the beds of streams nearly dried up in summer (and) natural and artificial ponds, preserved or made, to afford an adequate supply of stock-water."*

He next examined the question of whether soil conditions are capable of producing an inorganic gas poison, the so-called 'malarial hypothesis'. Drake first acknowledges the difficulty of characterizing the *"earthy surface"* of any area. Nowhere in *"our Valley"* does there exist any surface that is nothing but the *"fragments and powder of the subjacent rocks, and the different salts, or oxides, formed by their decomposition, under the influence of heat, water, and atmospheric air."* All rocky strata have crumbled and have become the *nidus* of some kind of plant. Decaying plant-matter added to the underpinning of mineral matter has prepared the spot for *"a vegetation of a higher order."* The appearance of pools, swamps, and running streams led to new plant and animal life as well as to the movement from one place to another of both organic and inorganic matter.

Having established the origin of the soil's complexity, he observed that (all other circumstances being equal):

> *The Fever prevails most where the organic matter is most abundant, in or resting on the soil; that where the surface is not moist enough to favor the decomposition of organic matter, the Fever has but little prevalence; that a temperature of sixty degrees of Fahrenheit, or above, is necessary to fermentation and putrefaction, and that the Fever ceases, in going north, when we reach a summer temperature below that degree; that particular localities have experienced the Fever, in an epidemic form, when a surface abounding in organic matter has been newly exposed to the action of the summer sun; and that under long condition, which exhausts the organic matter of the soil, and prevents its accumulation on the surface, the Fever almost ceases to appear.*

None of these facts, he argued, prove the existence of malaria-causing gas. The gases that are known to be produced, e.g. carbonic acid, carbonic oxide, carbureted hydrogen, have not been shown to produce autumnal fever. Finally, arguing by analogy:

> *The assumed undiscovered gas, called malaria, must be of the same character; and, therefore, at all times and places be productive of the same effects. Now, although autumnal fever is a disease of intrinsic uniformity, it shows modifications which have not been explained by the assignment of modifying causes; and without such causes, its diversities constitute an objection to the existence of a single agent of an unchangeable character.*

Drake addressed last the 'vegeto-animalcular' hypothesis, which ascribes autumnal fever "*to living organic forms, too small to be seen with the naked eye; and which may belong either to the vegetable or animal kingdom, or partake of the characters of both.*" No less than 14 observations are made in favor of this hypothesis, beginning with what the microscope has uncovered, namely "*the existence of countless variety of organic forms.*" By imagining each form living off of forms smaller in size, a point is reached where "*living, organic forms, both animal and vegetable, may be of such size, as to float permanently in the air.*"

The next observations are all based on reasoning by analogy. The existence of poisonous creatures suggested that microscopic animals or plants might similarly be harmful. Since the southern regions are where the most poisonous animals and plants are located, one might suppose that "*the microscopic beings in those regions are more pernicious than those of higher latitudes."* All living matter needs water, so dependence on water probably extends to *"the tribes that are invisible."* Similarly, high temperature is probably favorable to *"the invisible"* since it is favorable to the development of animal and vegetable life. Decomposition favors growth in the visible world, as it probably does for the *"myriads of microscopic beings (that) swarm around."*

The close resemblance of larger plants and animals suggested the presence of *"two distinct species of the same natural order of microscopic beings"* that produce autumnal fever, one the cause of intermittents, the other of remittents - diversities that are *"inexplicable on the malarial hypothesis."* The vegeto-animacular hypothesis also had the advantage of explaining the delay between exposure to and outbreak of disease, since many poisons are known to take some time before they develop their effects.

The variability of the autumnal fevers from year to year is analogous to the fact that a year *"of great abundance may be followed by one unproductive."* Furthermore

> *It has often happened, that musquitoes (sic) have been absent, from the banks of the middle portion of the Ohio river, for a year and in the next appeared in immense numbers. We have but to suppose insect forms of a parallel size, to live under corresponding laws, and the hypothesis now before us, offers an explanation of sickly and healthy seasons.*

Drake was neither the first nor the last to consider that the quality of the soil played an important part in the epidemiology of malaria. In 1797, Samuel L. Mitchell, while undertaking a geological and mineral survey of New York State, hypothesized the presence of some sort of relationship between the different kinds of soils or rock strata of a region and the *"septic exhalations"* that were thought to be the cause of fevers and epidemic diseases. Furthermore, it is clear from Drake's own account that physicians he met during his travels shared his belief that the soil was one of the more important factors to take into account when reviewing the epidemic qualities of any region. Alphonse Laveran, who discovered the malaria parasite in 1880, accepted that malaria was linked one way or another with the soil. Hirsch, writing in 1886, noted that *"there are, indeed, few points in the etiology upon which observers are so agreed, as that the soil has an influence in the production of malaria."*

Drake was also not the first to realize that malaria was often present in areas that were devoid of swamps and marshes. The importance of some water, was such, however, as to lead later in the century, especially in Italy and

France, to a malaria version of Pettenkofer's cholera ground-water theory. This theory was particularly strong during the decades immediately before Ross' discovery of the mosquito's role in the transmission of malaria. Hirsch presented it in the following terms:

> *It can be shown that the intensity of the morbific influence is materially increased by the porosity and hygroscopic character of the soil; and accordingly the alluvial and diluvial formations are classical ground for malaria, while the older formations are more or less exempt in proportion to the compactness of the rock.*

According to Corrado Tommasi-Crudeli, an Italian scientist, malaria was caused by a *"living ferment, which finds conditions favorable to its existence and its multiplications in soils of the most different natures."* It was not necessary to the production of the disease; only a small amount of humidity in the immediate subsoil is sufficient, if the earth contains the "germs of the ferment." Sufficiently humid, malarious earth allows the ferment to pass into the atmosphere where it can be breathed. This theory also fitted well with the generally well-accepted fact that malarious fevers often increased when the soil was disturbed.

In 1879 Tommasi-Crudeli and Edwin Klebs (1834-1913) announced that they had found the cause of malaria. The "living ferment" was, in fact, a bacterium (*Bacillus malariae*). For several years they argued that Laveran's parasites were merely products of degeneration of red blood cells. Other investigators added fungi to the list of possible non-miasmic causes of malaria.

Despite multiple claims to the contrary, A.-F. Dubergé, in his book *Le Paludisme* published in 1895, noted that up until then, *"no microorganisms had been found either in the soil, water or air, that could be attributed a specific role in malaria."* He too assigned *"feverish soil"* as the leading cause of malaria. For the moment, the malaria parasite had only been found in the blood of malarious patients. That mosquitoes transmitted the parasite from human to human would shortly be discovered (1898).

What is striking in this history is how little the 'germ' nature of malaria altered thinking concerning its transmission. Miasmatic emanations had been replaced with ferments or microbes floating in the air. Both miasmas and microbes could enter the human body via the lungs, or conceivably they could penetrate the skin and enter the blood stream directly. What is also striking, however, is how close the explanations were to implicating mosquitoes. All of Drake's text fully supports the role of the mosquito as the transmitter of the malaria parasite.

Epidemic Puerperal Fever - A Hand or An Air Borne Disease?

None of those things cause the (puerperal fever) epidemic; it is the nursing and medical staff who carry the microbe from an infected woman to a healthy one ... (Pasteur, 1879)

Slightly less than 90 years before an exasperated Louis Pasteur (1822-1896) strode to the blackboard to draw the bacillus responsible for puerperal fever, the Scottish physician Alexander Gordon (1752-1799) concluded, during Aberdeen's 1789-92 epidemic, that puerperal fever was a *"specific contagion or infection"* transmitted from one patient to another by a third party (midwife, nurse or himself). Gordon, who had trained earlier at Edinburgh and Leiden, and who may have been Aberdeen's only trained obstetrician at the time, came to this conclusion after a careful analysis of some 77 patients affected with the fever that he had attended at the Aberdeen Dispensary. Also, by observing that the epidemic prevailed in the new town and not in the old town of Aberdeen, he was able to conclude that *"the mystery is explained, when I inform the reader that the midwife, Mrs Jeffries, who had all the practice of that town, was so very fortunate as not to fall in with the infection; otherwise the women whom she delivered would have shared the fate of others."*

Observing that these two towns were only one mile apart, and that often the fever would strike one ward in a clinic and not others, allowed Gordon to conclude - *"the cause of the epidemic ... was not owing to a noxious constitution of the atmosphere."* Gordon was not, however, able to determine the exact means whereby the infection was carried by the *"third party."* He adopted the methods recommended by the *"excellent author,"* the *"ingenious Dr. (James) Lind (for the) purification of infected chambers, and for the fumigation of infected apparel,"* to which Gordon added

> *the patient's apparel and bedclothes ought either to be burnt or thoroughly purified; and the nurses and physicians who have attended patients affected with puerperal fever ought carefully to wash themselves, and to get their apparel properly fumigated before it be put on again.*

Holmes, who publicly recognized Gordon's contributions, was the first American physician to call puerperal fever a contagion. In 1843 he published an essay entitled *The contagiousness of puerperal fever*, which had as its main object to show that "*the disease ... is so far contagious as to be frequently carried from patient to patient by physicians and nurses.*" He even went so far in his public statements as to declare that "*doctors were instruments of death*" and that they should clean their hands and clothes. His conclusions were drawn from case histories found in earlier British literature. In at least twenty of these cases, Holmes had noted that the physicians of patients who contracted the disease had earlier examined patients with puerperal fever or performed autopsies on persons who had died from it.

Holmes did not conclude that doctor to patient was the only means whereby puerperal fever could be transmitted. This was but one means, one which he qualified with a "*sometimes*" or "*frequently.*" Following the then dominant thinking concerning the cause of puerperal fever, Holmes "*granted that the disease may be produced and variously modified by many causes besides contagion, and more especially by epidemic and endemic influences.*" He believed, for example, as an "*undisputed fact that within the walls of lying-in hospitals there is often generated a miasma, palpable as the chlorine used to destroy it, tenacious so as in some cases almost to defy extirpation, deadly in some institutions as the plague.*"

Epidemic influences on puerperal fever invariably were seen to involve miasmatic or atmospheric factors, while endemic influences included these and many other possibilities, as can be seen from the following text taken from an 1845 medical publication on the subject:

> to difficult labour; to inflammation of the uterus; to accumulation of noxious humors, set in motion by labour; to violent mental emotion, stimulants, and obstructed perspiration; to miasmata, admission of cold air to the body, and into the uterus; to hurried circulation; to suppression of lacteal secretion; diarrhoea; liability to putrid contagion from changes in the humors during pregnancy; hasty separation of the placenta; binding the abdomen too tight; sedentary employment; stimulating or spare diet; or to fashionable dissipation.

Ignaz Semmelweis (1809-1865) may have been the first to argue that **every** case of puerperal fever was due to its direct transfer from the attending doctor, nurse or midwife. In 1847 Semmelweis became responsible for supervising the maternity clinic in Vienna where obstetricians were trained. Midwives were trained in another clinic. Semmelweis noted that the incidence of puerperal fever in that clinic for the previous several years had been about three times less than in his clinic. Commissions that had investigated the disparity had concluded that the disease was epidemic and thus beyond control, leading Semmelweis to sarcastically note

against childbed (puerperal) fever that is due to atmospheric, cosmic, terrestrial influences there can be no defense. The advocates of an epidemic theory secure themselves behind this indefensibility; they thereby escape all responsibility for the devastations of the disease.

Tabelle Nr. XVII.

Standesausweis der k. k. Gebäranstalt vom 16. August 1784 angefangen.

Jahr	Aufge- nommen	Zahl der Gestor- benen	Percent- Antheil	Jahr	Aufge- nommen	Zahl der Gestor- benen	Percent- Antheil
1784	284	6	2,11	1817	2735	25	0,91
1785	890	13	1,44	1818	2568	56	2,18
1786	1151	5	0,43	1819	3089	154	4,98
1787	1407	5	0,35	1820	2998	75	2,50
1788	1425	5	0,35	1821	3294	55	1,66
1789	1246	7	0,56	1822	3066	26	0,84
1790	1326	10	0,75	1823	2872	214	7,45
1791	1395	8	0,57	1824	2911	144	4,94
1792	1574	14	0,89	1825	2594	229	4,82
1793	1684	44	2,61	1826	2359	192	8,12
1794	1768	7	0,39	1827	2367	51	2,15
1795	1798	38	2,11	1828	2833	101	3,56
1796	1904	22	1,16	1829	3012	140	4,64
1797	2012	5	0,24	1830	2797	111	3,97
1798	2046	5	0,24	1831	3353	222	6,62
1799	2067	20	0,96	1832	3331	105	3,15
1800	2070	41	1,98	1833	3907	205	5,25
1801	2106	17	0,80	1834	4218	355	8,41
1802	2346	9	0,38	1835	4040	227	5,61
1803	2215	16	0,72	1836	4144	331	7,98
1804	2022	8	0,39	1837	4363	375	8,59
1805	2112	9	0,40	1838	4560	179	3,92
1806	1875	13	0,69	1839	4992	248	4,96
1807	925	6	0,63	1840	5166	328	6,44
1808	855	7	0,81	1841	5454	330	6,05
1809	912	13	1,42	1842	6024	730	12,11
1810	744	6	0,80	1843	5914	457	7,72
1811	1050	20	1,90	1844	6244	336	5,38
1812	1419	9	0,63	1845	6756	313	4,63
1813	1945	21	1,08	1846	7027	567	8,06
1814	2062	66	3,20	1847	7039	210	2,68
1815	2591	19	0,73	1848	7095	91	1,28
1816	2410	12	0,49				

Convinced that puerperal fever could not be of miasmatic origin, Semmelweis began his studies to determine what was its cause. A critical moment in his investigations was the death of a colleague who had died from injuries incurred while dissecting a corpse. Upon dissecting his colleagues' body, Semmelweis recognized pathological states similar to those he had seen in women who had died of puerperal fever. He reasoned that the cause of death was the same. The death of his colleague was known to be the introduction of decaying matter into his blood stream; puerperal fever was, therefore, due to the introduction of such matter in the uterus of pregnant women. It also followed that puerperal fever and pyaemia (blood poison-ing) were but two forms of the same disease. Semmelweis believed that this disease arose from some form of chemically driven fermentation or putrefaction, along the lines proposed by Justus von Liebig (1803-73), a German chemist, a position that Pasteur would later attack.

In 1848, Semmelweis introduced hand washing in his clinic. All doctors were required to wash in a chlorine solution until the skin was slippery and the cadaver smell was gone. Striking results were quickly realized. Within one month the rates were below those of the midwives' clinics. Semmelweis' conclusions were published in editorials written by supportive colleagues. At the same time, he and his friends wrote to other clinics announcing their discovery and inviting comments. The general response was favorable, except for the sentiment that puerperal fever could also be caused by other means. Most respondents still favored the traditional miasmatic or atmospheric influences. Also, there remained the sentiment that Semmelweis had not fully proved his case, leading one critic to advise:

> If adoption of the washings makes it possible to avoid even the least significant of the many concurring factors that cause puerperal fever, then (Semmelweis') was a sufficient large service. However, whether this is in fact the case, only a later time will be able to decide. In the meantime, I believe we should wait and wash.

Semmelweis' term of appointment came to an end in mid 1849. He had yet to publish his findings in detail, and it seems that his difficult personality had made him unpopular with the administration and many of his colleagues. When only offered a minor re-appointment, one that would not allow him to continue his research, he left Vienna in 1850 to return to his home in Budapest. Carl Braun, who disliked Semmelweis intensely, succeeded him.

Braun wrote extensively on puerperal fever. In his first major piece, written in 1855, he listed thirty possible causes, of which the 28th was *"cadaver infection."* He shunned Semmelweis' theory of chlorine disinfection, but in his practice required that any student whose hands smelled of a corpse would not be permitted to examine a woman in labor!

Braun, unlike Semmelweis, expressed interest in the possibility that puerperal fever was caused by a microorganism. Braun was aware of the work of Jacob Henle (1809-1885), a German pathologist and anatomist, concerning contagion. In an 1840 publication *On miasmata and contagia* Henle formulated the hypothesis that *"the material of contagion is not only organic but living, endowed with individual life and standing to the diseased body in the relation of a parasitic organism."* Such living agents, *contagioum vivum*, were responsible for the second and third categories of the three groups of diseases he recognized:

Plague Legends

1. those that are miasmatic and not, so far as is known, contagious, of which malaria is the only example;
2. those that arise as miasmatic diseases but are also spread by contagion (e.g. smallpox, typhus, influenza, cholera, plague);
12.those that are contagious and not miasmatic (e.g. syphilis).

He suggested that the living agent was given off from the body of the sick and capable of producing the same disease in others.[68] For the second group, the agent is diffused through the atmosphere, while for the third group, it is via material objects, e.g. those soiled with pus. Also, he imagined that healthy individuals could be the *"carriers of the infectious material which may be attached to them externally."*

Armed with Henle's conjecture, Braun favored the possibility that the epidemic cases of puerperal fever were caused by germs conveyed through the air into the open wounds of maternity patients. He observed that this was a new materialistic interpretation of the old concept of a miasma.

In 1860, several years after Braun's most recent publication on the subject, Semmelweis finally published his main book *The Etiology, the Concept, and the Prevention of Puerperal Fever*. Much of the book is a polemic against his detractors, including Braun, whose ideas Semmelweis categorically dismissed. Again most reviewers accepted Semmelweis' position that the absorption of decaying animal-organic matter can cause puerperal fever but as before they disagreed that it was the only way the infection could be transmitted. Most obstetricians still believed in multiple causes for puerperal fever, including Braun's air-borne one.

The 'hand' borne and bacterial basis of puerperal fever received confirmation in the results of studies carried out by Carl Mayrhofer (1837-1882), one of Braun's assistants. Appointed in 1862 and initially actively encouraged by Braun, Mayrhofer sought to find microorganisms in the uterine discharges from puerperal fever victims. He, like Braun, was familiar with Henle's conjecture; he was also familiar with Pasteur's conclusion that fermentation was always due to living ferments. He was thus fully prepared to look for living forms in his studies.

---

[68] Henle was influenced by Agostino Bassi's (1773-1856) demonstration in 1836 that a specific fungus caused muscadine, a disease of silk-worms. By 1840 several other instances of *contagium vivum* had been demonstrated.

From an examination of the discharges from more than one hundred women Mayrhofer found one form that was most abundant and regularly present. He injected these 'vibrions' into the genitals of newly delivered rabbits; the rabbits invariably became diseased and died. Post-mortem examination revealed morbid changes similar to those in humans who had died of puerperal fever. These results were published in the period 1863-65. In the 1865 paper Mayrhofer observed that, while the harmful material that caused puerperal fever could be conveyed through the air, infection was usually due to the *"examining finger."*

Mayrhofer's 1865 publication was essentially his last on the subject, while that of Braun was an 1881 publication in which, despite the investigations of Mayrhofer and others, and in total contradiction with Pasteur's position, he still insisted that infection usually occurred through the air, and was not bacterial in origin but instead toxic dried vegetable organisms. Braun was not alone in his beliefs, as is evident from the 1879 incident that led Pasteur to accuse the nursing and medical staff of carrying deadly microbes from sick to healthy women (see opening quote).

Pasteur was provoked by the presentation of the academician, Hervieux who contrasted the true *"miasm or puerperal fever"* with *"those microorganisms which are widely distributed in nature, and which, after all, appear fairly inoffensive, since we constantly live in their midst without being thereby disturbed."* When Hervieux reacted to Pasteur's accusation by saying that no one would ever find this microbe, Pasteur darted to the blackboard replying - There, that is what it is like! - after drawing organisms shaped like strings of beads, now known under the name of 'streptococcus'.[69]

Gordon was driven from his post in 1795 soon after he published his essay concerning puerperal fever and he never practiced obstetrics again. Holmes was violently opposed by his obstetrical colleagues. Semmelweis ended his life in an insane asylum. Mayrhofer turned to morphine and died at the early age of 45. Despite all of the constraints faced by these and other investigators,

---

[69] The day after their confrontation, Hervieux invited Pasteur to see a woman gravely ill with puerperal fever. Blood was taken from her finger from which Pasteur was able to cultivate a microorganism similar to those that he had found in the pus of abscesses in 1875. After her death several days later, he was able to cultivate the same microorganism from the pus taken from her abdominal cavity.

however, their work set the foundation upon which Pasteur and others would build the new age of microbiology, an age to which we turn next.

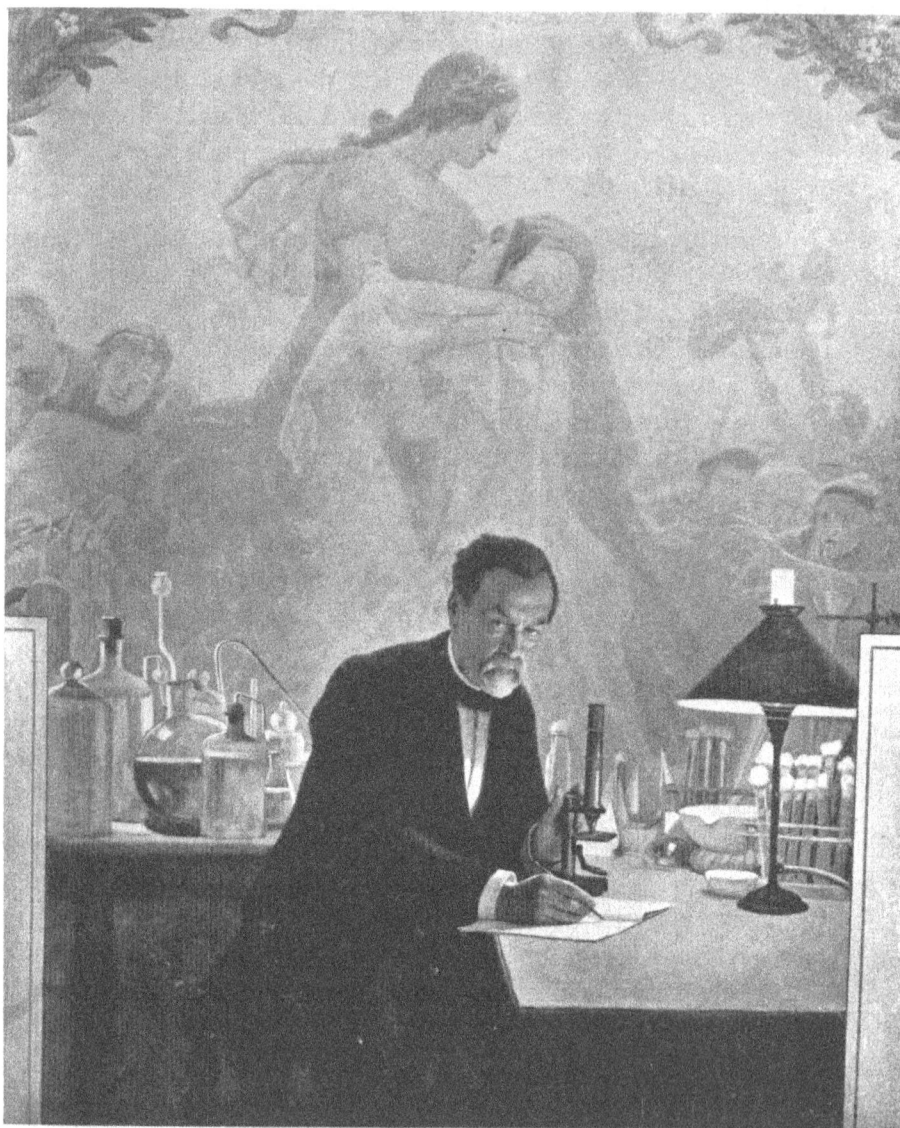

L.-ED. FOURNIER.

La Science et l'Humanité.
Décoration dans l'ancien laboratoire de Pasteur, à l'École Normale de Paris (fragment). (Cliché Braun.)

Pasteur Takes on Spontaneous Generation

He that thoroughly understands the nature of ferments and fermentations, shall probably be much better able than he that ignores them, to give a fair account of divers phenomena of several diseases (as well fevers as others) which will perhaps be never thoroughly understood, without an insight into the doctrine of fermentation. (Boyle, 1663)

The possibility that life could arise from putrefying organic matter seems to have been accepted early in history. It was so common an observation that not to believe in 'spontaneous generation' was to deny the obvious. Aristotle, and later Harvey, Descartes, Boyle and Newton, all accepted it without serious question. The Royal Society in one of its early sessions even met to explore whether insects could be made from cheese as some claimed!

Many attempts were made before Pasteur to disprove that life could arise out of dead matter, and as would happen to Pasteur, non-believers would counter with new evidence forcing yet another cycle of experimentation. One such cycle was started by Francesco Redi (1626-98), an Italian physician, who attacked the problem by showing that pieces of meat, which normally would 'give rise' to maggots when exposed to the air in hot weather, did not when the jar within which they lay was covered with a fine piece of gauze. The gauze was not fine enough to keep out fine particles in the air, but it did keep away the flies out of whose eggs maggots would arise. Redi concluded from this experiment that no form of living matter could arise from dead organic matter.

To disprove Redi's conclusions, John T. Needham (1713-81), an English clergyman of the catholic faith, repeated the experiment but this time using chicken broth, which he bottled, boiled, corked, re-heated and cooled.[70] Upon finding the 'animalcules' of Leeuwenhoek in the broth, Needham concluded that they had appeared spontaneously. Convinced that Needham had failed to protect his infusion from the air, Lazzaro Spallanzani (1729-99), an Italian Abbé, modified the experiment by using flasks with slender necks which were sealed off while the flasks were immersed in boiling water so that both the liquid and the air above it were completely protected against

---

[70] Needham was the first clergyman of his faith to become a member of the Royal Society of London (1768).

contamination from without. No microorganisms were found in the broth. Proponents of spontaneous generation responded that he had only proved that spontaneous generation could not occur without air!

The controversy was again renewed in the 19th century by which time it was understood that oxygen was needed for the life process. By now the recipes for generating spontaneously mice and insects had totally given way to the search for Leeuwenhoek's animaculae. Experiments, carried out in 1836 and 1837 by German scientists in which oxygen was present, again showed negative results, and again believers in spontaneous generation argued that the conditions of the experiment, notwithstanding the presence of oxygen, were not compatible with the generation of living matter.

Matters became even more complicated when in the 1850s several experimenters, who themselves were antagonistic to spontaneous generation, had such great difficulty in protecting milk and egg yolk from putrefaction that they were forced to conclude that the germs of putrefaction came from the substances themselves and were derived from animal tissues.

It was around this time that Pasteur was deeply involved in his studies of fermentation. As conjectured by Boyle in the 17th century (see quote above), understanding fermentation was a key piece to the disease puzzle. Contrary to Liebig, however, who was taking a line well familiar to Boyle and the other iatrochemists of his time, Pasteur believed that fermentation, instead of being a strictly chemical process, had to be one in which a living form was involved. While his first investigations concerned alcoholic fermentation, his first major publication dealt with lactic acid fermentation. This was in 1857. Already in this publication he set out the principle, which would prove essential to his later work concerning disease microbes, namely that each different type of fermentation corresponded to a different ferment. He knew that his conclusions went beyond the established facts. He said so much at the end of his memoir, when he noted "*I have taken my stand unreservedly in an order of ideas which, strictly speaking, cannot be irrefutably demonstrated.*"

By 1859 Pasteur had so mastered the laboratory techniques involved that he could bring about almost at will one or another type of fermentation and to determine what had caused it. In one such experiment the causative agent proved to be a motile microorganism. At first, Pasteur hesitated to accept this result because motility was thought to be an attribute limited to animal life and at that time it was thought that ferments had to be a form of plant life. He called these motile agents 'infusoria', deliberately adopting a vague word since any more definitive name would be *"arbitrary"* and amount to adopting *"definite rules of nomenclature for organisms that can be differentiated only by characteristics of which we do not know the true significance."*

One such characteristic was the ability of his 'infusoria' to live without air. He discovered this attribute when on looking down the microscope he saw them immobile at the edge of the lens covering the liquid they were in, while those in the center were moving actively. They seemed to want to move to the center away from the oxygen. He designated life that needed oxygen with the word 'aerobic' and life without oxygen 'anaerobic'. He correctly guessed that anaerobic life was dependent on the presence of other microscopic germs that used up the oxygen in the surrounding medium. He went on to think, without any immediate experimentation, that it was exactly this kind of process that was involved in the phenomena of putrefaction. The foul odor associated with decomposition of beef bouillon, egg albumin, or meat is the result of the anaerobic life of specialized germs that attack proteins under the oxygen-removing protection of aerobic life. A short time later, after his experiments concerning spontaneous generation, he concluded that - 1. true fermentation depends upon … microscopic organisms, 2. these organisms do not have a spontaneous origin, 3. life in the absence of oxygen is concomitant with fermentation.

As noted above, Pasteur's conclusions were in total opposition to those of Liebig who, working with animal tissues, such as liver and muscle, conjectured in 1842 that diseases were caused by a chemical action instigated by a decomposing substance coming in contact with living cells. This process had its parallel in fermentation arising from yeast. Inside the body, instead of yeast, there was some unknown ingredient that when present would allow disease poisons to multiply by chemical, not biological, means. This came to be known as the 'zymotic' theory of disease.

The zymotic theory of disease was furthered by the work of Rudolph Virchow (1821-1902), who took pathological investigations one level lower than where Bichat had left it, i.e. to the level of the cell. Virchow deemed germ theory *"superficial."* He believed that diseases came from abnormal changes within cells. He even developed a 'neo-humoralism' which held that abnormal changes originated in an imbalance of protein substances in the blood. He opposed for years the ideas of Semmelweis concerning puerperal fever. He correctly concluded, however, that Würzburg, where he had been professor of pathology, was free of cholera due to the purity of its water-supply system, a position that Pettenkofer opposed, for reasons discussed earlier.[71]

Pasteur's investigations concerning fermentation had reached the point where it became of critical importance to demonstrate once and for all where did the 'infinitely small' come from. Furthermore, having linked together germs, putrefaction and contagious diseases, it logically followed that he was obliged to enter the controversy on spontaneous generation.

A perfect opportunity was provided Pasteur when the Academy instituted in 1860 the Alhumbert Prize with the objective - *"To attempt, by carefully conducted experiments, to throw new light on the question of the so-called spontaneous generations."* The Academy had decided to offer this prize following a paper read by Félix Archimède Pouchet before the Paris Academy of Sciences, in which he claimed to have produced spontaneous generation. Pouchet was director of the Museum of Natural History in Rouen, and a member of many learned societies.

Pouchet's experiment consisted of taking a flask of boiling water, which was hermetically sealed, and then plunging it upside down into a basin of mercury. After the water had become cold, he opened the flask under mercury and introduced half a liter of oxygen and a small quantity of hay infusion previously exposed for a long time to a very high temperature. Within a few days, microbial growth regularly appeared in the hay infusion.

Before embarking on his own experiments, Pasteur wrote the following to Pouchet:

> *I think you are wrong, not in believing in spontaneous generation (for it is difficult in such a case not to have a preconceived idea), but in affirming the existence of spontaneous generation. In experimental science it is always a mistake not to doubt when facts do not compel affirmation ... In my opinion, the question is whole and untouched by decisive proofs.*

Systematically Pasteur discovered the error in all of the experiments then purporting to demonstrate spontaneous generation. He showed that mercury invariably contained dust and living germs on its surface. He found that it

---

[71] Later, in the 1860s and 1870s, when the public health movement in Germany was undergoing rapid development, Virchow championed sewage disposal, especially in Berlin. He made Berlin a healthy city, as Pettenkofer had Munich.

was necessary to heat eggs and milk to higher temperatures to eliminate any germs they may contain. There still remained, however, the problem of how to conduct the experiment in the presence of ordinary air without contaminating the sterile matter under study. The solution was the use of the swanneck flask, a flask that had been introduced in Pasteur's laboratory by another investigator. Such a flask is made by drawing the neck of a heated flask into the form of a sinuous S-tube.

Pasteur proceeded to make many such flasks after first placing a fermentable fluid in their insides. The liquid was boiled for a few minutes, the vapor forcing out the air through the narrow orifice of the neck. The outside air returned while the flask slowly cooled. He found that the fluid remained sterile indefinitely. The wet walls of the neck trapped whatever germs had entered the flask before they could reach the infusion. That the infusion itself was capable of supporting microscopic life was shown by breaking the neck, allowing dust to fall on its surface, and watching it appear, first at the spot directly under the opening. This simple apparatus left the opposition without any argument, although it did not prevent Pouchet from publishing later in 1864 a new and larger edition of his earlier book on the subject!

Armed with such an apparatus, Pasteur and his collaborators were able to demonstrate the uneven distribution of the germs of putrefaction and fermentation. For this it was necessary to seal the flask with the aid of a blowpipe and then break the neck very carefully where measurements were to be made. The flasks were resealed after air had entered them and placed in an incubator for later evaluation. In this way, they found that aerial germs were most abundant in low places, especially near cultivated earth, while those opened in the midst of the Swiss glaciers remained sterile.

In 1862 the Academy awarded Pasteur the Prix Alhumbert for his *Mémoires sur les corpuscles organisés qui existent dans l'atmosphere....* Pasteur, in a lecture delivered in 1864, in which he described these experiments, concluded - "*Life is a germ and a germ is Life. Never will the doctrine of spontaneous generation recover from the mortal blow of this simple experiment.*"

Pasteur was well aware that his arguments against spontaneous generation would have encountered less suspicion if he were not a pious catholic. But it was his strong belief in God that contributed to his assault on this ancient belief. If living organisms could emerge from dead matter - "*God as author of life would then no longer be needed.*" While he realised that he could not prove that spontaneous generation was impossible, his faith pushed him to demonstrate that all experiments purporting to have demonstrated spontaneous generation were wrong.

That the 'infinitely small' was the cause and not the result of fermentation and putrefaction forced a radical rethinking of the origin of disease. That each specific minute living form was responsible for a specific form of fermentation paralleled the argument made earlier by Bretonneau that the specificity of disease was due to the specificity of cause. Thus, disease specificity and germ specificity were logically linked by the work of Pasteur well before he, himself, entered the arena of human diseases.

That the assault on spontaneous generation occurred at the same time that the microbial basis of epidemic diseases was being established was no accident. Belief in spontaneous generation supported the non-specificity of diseases, as well as the internal, pathological origin and development of disease. Such a belief obviated the need to call upon any external disease-causing agents; whatever living matter was found in the sick was a consequence of putrefaction and fermentation. Such a belief had given rise to the notion of 'laudable' pus, a notion that over the centuries many surgeons had held for centuries.[72] Pasteur demonstrated just the opposite; he turned the whole issue around. Now it remained to find which living forms were responsible for which diseases, and to demonstrate that no other forms were involved, a simple sounding proposition but one which has proved in the event to be much more difficult than anyone could possibly have imagined.

---

[72] Even the great Joseph Lister, who was inspired by the results of Pasteur to introduce antiseptic surgery beginning in 1865, believed that the pus in an unopened abscess was, as a rule, free of microorganisms. He thought pus to be sterile and not subject to putrefaction until it came into contact with microorganisms in the air after the abscess was opened. He was still arguing this position in 1881.

The Disease Causation Postulates of Koch

The study of germs offers so many connections with the diseases of animals and plants, that it certainly constitutes a first step in the ... serious investigation of putrid and contagious diseases. (Pasteur)

When Henle conjectured in 1840 that microorganisms might cause many diseases, he did not rule out other causes for the same disease condition. Henle did, however, address a question that was of essential importance to advancing the case for the microbial basis for disease, namely, how could one prove that microbes, as they would eventually be called, caused disease. He, himself, was rather skeptical that such a proof could be realized. He visualized the key problem was that of isolating *"the contagious organisms from the contagious fluids, and then observ(ing) the powers of each separately."*

Henle's criterion required that one locate and isolate individual microbes, and then confirm that they did indeed cause disease. This was the first of several postulates that would be further developed by Koch some forty years later. In the late 1860s several researchers reported identifying microorganisms in specific disease processes. One of them was Mayrhofer, as discussed earlier; another was Klebs. Mayrhofer addressed puerperal fever, Klebs the problem of infection arising from gunshot wounds.

In a series of papers, Klebs addressed Henle's question of proof. In 1872 he observed that *"tracing the invasion and the course of the microorganisms can make causality probable, but the crucial experiment is to isolate the efficient cause and allow it to operate on the organism."* Here a second possible postulate has been added, namely, one of correlating the advancing parasites with the sequence of morbid changes. In the course of his studies, Klebs, a student of pathological anatomy, became more and more critical of his mentors, and at one point noted - *"Henle recognized, as the causes of disease, only universal physical and chemical influences, the life impulses, the same factors that have often been identified by others who wrote before and after him. The concept of a specific cause of a disease, which is absolutely destructive of life, is alien to him as to most other pathologists."* It should be noted, however, that Klebs identified a number of 'specific causes' that were grossly in error, such as the malaria parasite in earth mentioned earlier.

Around this time Koch was studying the etiology of anthrax, a cattle disease that his studies would show to be caused by the specific bacillus, *Bacillus anthracis.* Koch learned that the mere presence of anthrax bacilli in an animal did not ensure that it would become diseased. So a strict cause and effect had to be ruled out.

However, by developing better inoculation techniques he was able to obtain higher fatality rates among the test animals. Following Henle, he also tried inoculating with anthrax substances that did not contain the bacilli. These invariably failed to cause disease. On the basis of these results, he concluded - *"anthrax never occurs without viable anthrax bacilli or spores. In my opinion no more conclusive proof can be given that anthrax bacilli are the true and only cause of anthrax."* His critics demanded that he separate the bacilli from associated substances, to which he replied *"this is impossible ... no one can take seriously such an undertaking."*

Koch then turned to the study of wound infections. In 1878, during these studies, he wrote that a conclusive proof of the parasitic origin of a disease *"would require that we find parasitic organisms in all cases of the disease, that they are present in such numbers and distribution that the disease symptoms can be explained, and that a morphologically distinguishable organism is identified for every different disease."* The latter clause is a new postulate, but in this formulation, it avoided the possible existence of morphologically *indistinguishable* organisms. In 1884, Koch acknowledged that morphological characteristics *"are not normally sufficient to distinguish bacteria,"* and in 1890, he insisted that every possible characteristic of different strains of organisms be considered before identifying them as the same species.

One theoretical obstacle that threatened the application of Koch's postulates was the erroneous belief that every bacterial species appeared in several morphological and physiological forms. Which form would be taken would depend on external conditions. The term 'pleomorphism' was introduced to describe the supposed change of bacteria from spherical cocci to bacillary rods to spirals. The doctrine of pleomorphism resulted in many workers being unaware that they were dealing with mixed cultures rather than a single specific agent, particularly when anaerobic agents were involved. It would not be until 1916 that cultures of anaerobic infections could be made easily and consistently.

In 1882 Koch announced the discovery of the tuberculosis bacillus. Earlier bacterial advances with animal borne as well as plant borne diseases had not caught the imagination of the public. Tuberculosis was different. Given its importance to human health, it is not surprising to learn that this announcement was received everywhere with great enthusiasm. Koch had

confronted innumerable technical problems in his laboratory before reaching
this result.

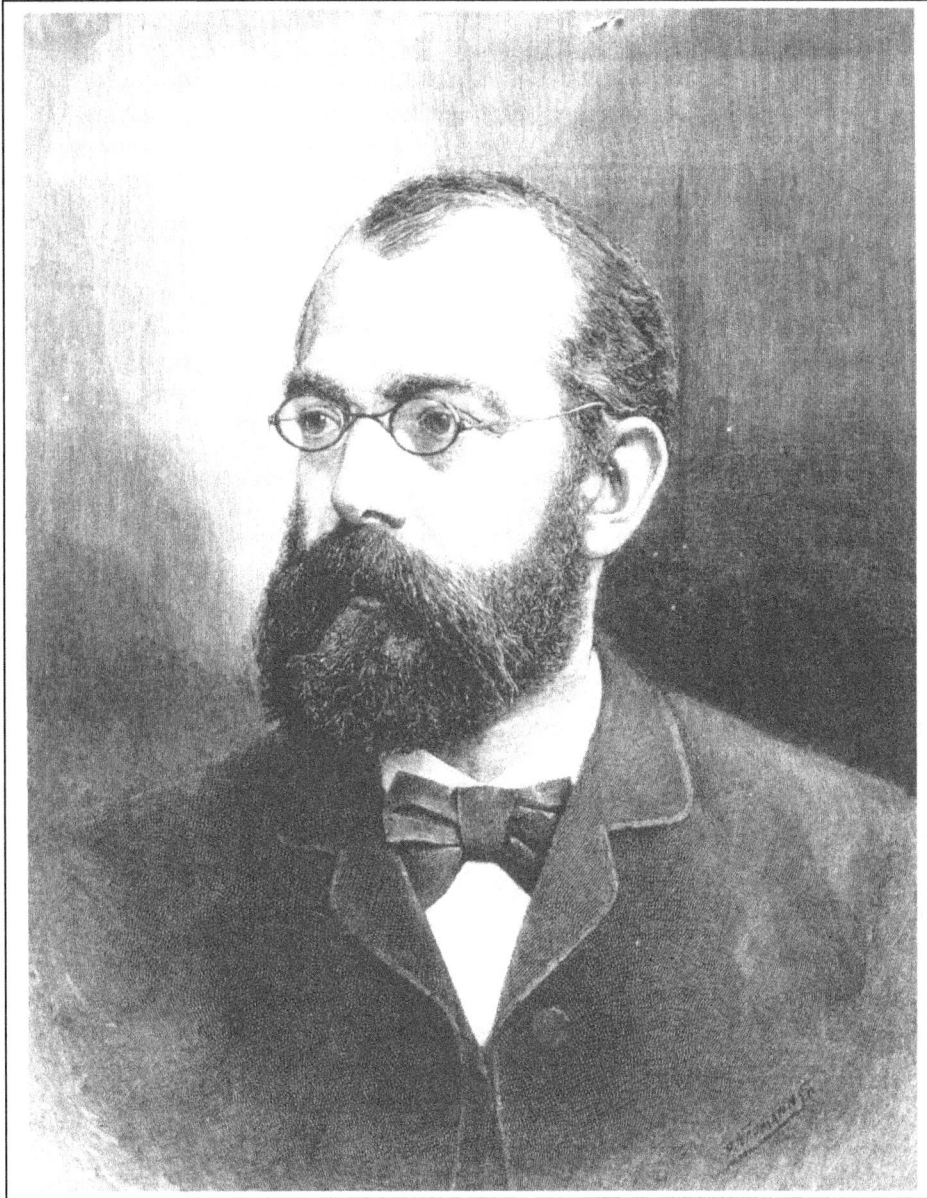

In the course of solving these problems, his ideas concerning disease causation matured considerably. His most complete statement on this question appeared in his 1884 paper on the etiology of tuberculosis:

> *First it is necessary to determine whether the diseased organs contain elements that are not constituents of the body or composed of such constituents. If such alien structures can be exhibited, it is necessary to determine whether they are organized and show signs of independent life. Such signs include motility - which is often confused with molecular motion - growth, propagation, and fructification. It is also necessary to consider the relation of such structures to their surroundings and to nearby tissues, their distribution in the body, their occurrence in various states of the disease, and so forth. Such considerations enable one to conclude that there is probably a causal connexion between the structures and the disease. Facts gained in these ways can provide so much evidence that only the most extreme sceptic would still object that the organisms may not be the cause, but only a concomitant of the disease. Often this objection has a certain justice, and, therefore, establishing the coincidence of the disease and the parasite is not conclusive. In addition, one requires a direct proof that the parasite is the actual cause. This can only be achieved by completely separating the parasites from the diseased organism and from all products of the disease that could be causally significant. If the isolated parasites are then introduced into healthy animals they must cause the disease with all its characteristics.*

This statement introduced new postulates, one, which Koch had previously thought impossible, namely the complete isolation of the parasite, the other, the demonstration that these isolated parasites, when inoculated in animals, cause the disease. It was his successful tuberculosis studies that had convinced him of the possibility and therefore of the necessity of isolating any supposed disease-causing agent and using pure isolates with experimental animals.

While it may seem most natural to seek microbes in sick patients, their presence in the natural environment, as demonstrated by Pasteur, led some to look for them there instead. For example, Klebs and Tommasi-Crudeli, as noted earlier, sought for, and thought that they had found the parasite that caused malaria in 'malarious earth'. Much earlier, in 1865, Pasteur participated in a commission that sought for the cholera germ in the air coming out of a hospital ward used for cholera patients. Their method was to fit a glass tube to the opening of the ward ventilators into which air would be drawn, in the hope that the poisonous agent would be caught in the condensation produced by the refrigeration mixture that surrounded the tube. Nothing incriminating was found.

The 1865 outbreak in Paris was the fourth cholera pandemic. It would be only during the next pandemic, which started in 1881, that cholera's bacterial cause would be discovered. When cholera broke out in Egypt in 1883, both France and Germany sent teams to investigate its cause. Koch, himself, headed the German team. While he searched for the invading organism in the tissues surrounding the intestinal lesions, the French team first attempted to reproduce the disease in animals. They could not succeed, since cholera is peculiarly a disease of man and animals do not have it. Tragically, Louis Ferdinand Thullier, one of Pasteur's assistants, caught cholera and died, causing the French team to return home.

Meanwhile the German team had seen bacteria in the intestine of cholera victims but had not isolated them or transmitted them to animals. Since the epidemic was nearing its end, they proceeded to Calcutta where the epidemic was still raging to continue their studies. There, 'vibrio comma', or as it would later be called, *Vibrio cholerae*, was isolated in pure culture. However, animal studies failed to reproduce the disease. No doubt the failure to provide conclusive proof contributed to Pettenkofer's stubborn position concerning the cause of cholera, as discussed earlier.

How difficult it was to satisfy Koch's postulates, as they would eventually come to be known, is seen in the history surrounding the false identification of a bacillus as the cause for influenza. Richard Pfeiffer, a colleague of Koch, and the head of the research department of Berlin's Institute for Infectious Diseases, first saw the bacillus that he claimed was the cause of influenza in the sputum of patients in the spring of 1890. His laboratory studies, however, did not begin until late 1891, after the peak of the epidemic had passed. He still found great quantities of the bacilli from patients with flu-like symptoms, and was able to raise the organism in pure culture. In search of a susceptible animal, he introduced the bacilli into mice, rats, guinea pigs, rabbits, monkeys, cats and dogs. Only the monkeys and rabbits fell ill. The monkeys became ill with a respiratory disease, which caused damaged to the lungs that reminded Pfeiffer of the lesions of influenza. The rabbits fell ill and even died, but their lesions were not typical of the disease. Despite these ambivalent results, Pfeiffer's bacillus, which later came to be known as *Haemophilus influenzae*, was largely accepted as the cause of influenza until it was displaced by influenza's true cause, a virus, which was isolated in the early 1930s.

An intriguing aspect of the influenza story is that *H. influenza* is needed along with the influenza virus to cause pigs to fall severely ill with what is known as swine flu. Had Pfeiffer used pigs to test his theory, it is conceivable that his bacterial cultures might have remained contaminated with the flu virus and that the pigs would have shown very typical flu-like lesions. Such results, although 'false', obviously would have solidified his claims.

Many other microbes proposed for one disease or another were quickly shown to be benign or agents of some other disease. For example, the bacillus isolated by Giuseppi Sanarelli, which he asserted to be that of yellow fever, proved to be the microbe of hog cholera. The search for microbes was so intense, that by 1884 one American medical leader was lamenting the 'bacteriomania' that had swept the medical profession. Physicians were 'discovering' and announcing new microbes each day, only to have to retract their results shortly thereafter.

Pasteur, himself, although he had contributed in a major way to confirming that anthrax was caused by the bacteria that Koch had discovered, approached the whole issue of disease causation differently. He and his co-workers turned their attention to the mechanisms of infection and immunity. Following the model used by Jenner to vaccinate against smallpox, Pasteur developed vaccines against chicken cholera and swine erysipelas.

Successful vaccination implicitly confirmed the causal nature of the agent used in the making of the vaccine. He then went on to develop a vaccine against rabies, a human disease, thereby breaking totally new grounds with spectacular and well-known results. His investigations also laid the foundation for a better understanding of immunity and the healthy carrier, both essential to the understanding of disease etiology.

Microbial Approach to Public Health

It will make no demonstrable difference in a city's mortality whether its streets are clean or not, whether the garbage is removed promptly or allowed to accumulate, or whether it has a plumbing law ... We can rest assured that however spick and span may be the streets ... as long as there is found the boor careless with his expectoration, and the doctor who cannot tell a case of polio from one of diphtheria, the latter disease, and tuberculosis

*as well, will claim their victims … Instead of an indiscriminate attack on
dirt, we must learn the nature and mode of transmission of each infection,
and must discover its most vulnerable point of attack. (Chapin)*

Charles V. Chapin (1856-1941) was wrong to argue that cleaning up the
environment would not improve human health. Nevertheless, this statement,
which comes from the beginning of the 20th century, no doubt reflected the
sentiments of some of the bacteriologists who, stimulated by the results of
Pasteur and Koch, began to uncover, one by one, the major scourges of
mankind.

As we have seen, public health initiatives of diverse kinds had been
introduced for a variety of reasons before the era of microbiology. Quarantine
measures were one of the earliest taken to prevent the spread of epidemic
disease. Initially aimed against the spread of plague, they were refined and
strengthened in the face of yellow fever and cholera. More often than not,
however, the medical community at best weakly supported these measures,
given their belief in the non-contagious nature of these and other diseases.

Other early initiatives were stimulated by the belief, as expressed by Mead,
that *"as nastiness is a great source of infection so cleanliness is the greatest
preventive."* Lind and Howard focussed on cleaning the air and rooms where
people were confined, in the (incorrect) belief that these would stop the
spread of typhus and typhoid. Initially confined to jails, ships, hospitals and
other closed institutions, these and other sanitary measures, became the
backbone of what came to be known as the 'sanitary movement'.

The sanitary movement, which had its roots in France and England in the
early part of the 19th century, was spurred by the continuing series of global
and regional epidemics that struck Europe and America, especially those of
cholera and yellow fever, which were particularly devastating in the overcrowded, poverty-ridden, dirty, and rapidly growing urban centres. The steps
taken to fight these diseases were mostly derived from non-contagionist
miasmatic concepts. In fact, medical belief in contagion receded and perhaps
reached its lowest point immediately before the studies of Pasteur and Koch.

Other motives for pushing for sanitary reforms of one kind or another
included humanitarian ones, which often had political overtones. When
Virchow, for example, participated as a medical officer in the review of the
typhus epidemic that was raging among the weavers in Upper Silesia in 1848,
he was already in opposition to the conservative leaders of Prussia. He took
this opportunity to attack the authorities of Berlin for having allowed

environmental conditions to develop that he felt were the root cause of the outbreak. His report focussed on the fact that authorities had not allowed autonomous self-rule, nor had they provided proper roads, nor agricultural and industrial improvements. From this point on, Virchow championed the cause of public health and social reform for the rest of his life.

The latter two decades of the 19th century saw the discovery of one disease-causing microbe after another. Of those discussed in this book, there were first the observations of the typhoid bacillus and the malaria parasite in 1880. Diphtheria (1884) followed those of tuberculosis (1882) and cholera (1883). Finally, in 1894, the plague bacterium was isolated. The role of the mosquito in the transmission of malaria and yellow fever was discovered in 1898 (bird malaria), 1899 (human malaria) and 1900 (yellow fever). The vectors of plague and typhus were only uncovered this century. The viral nature of influenza was not unraveled until the early 1930s, as mentioned earlier.

These developments altered the manner of combating disease, in some instances rather quickly, in others somewhat less so. Diphtheria, yellow fever, cholera and plague illustrate how knowledge gained by the new science of bacteriology was put into practical use.

Diphtheria

In 1871 M.J. Oertel produced false membranes in rabbits by swabbing their throats with membranous exudates obtained from human cases of diphtheria, and proved that the lesions were caused by a living agent by passing purulent matter through a series of six rabbits with each developing a false membrane. Since microscopic examination of the human membranes showed up many different living forms, he could not know which was the actual agent of the disease. In 1875 Klebs reported having found two kinds of agents in human diphtheric membranes, one a fungus, the other a bacillus. He failed to follow up these results and it was left to Friedrich Löffler, working in Koch's laboratory, to develop new culturing techniques and to announce in 1884 that Klebs' bacillus was indeed the cause of diphtheria. In one study, aimed at confirming his results, he attempted to culture the bacillus from the throats of twenty apparently healthy children, and much to his surprise, found one positive culture, which proved virulent for guinea pigs. This was the first bacteriological confirmation of a healthy human carrier of disease.

Two French bacteriologists, Emile Roux (1853-1933) and Alexandre Yersin (1863-1943), working at the newly established Pasteur Institute in Paris, confirmed Löffler's results and went on to isolate the poison that was conjectured to be the cause of paralyses associated with diphtheria. To get rid of the living baccili they forced the culture through a filter of fine unglazed porcelain. The clear filtrate, when injected into animals, caused all of the manifestations of the disease except the false membranes.

The next development took place in Koch's laboratory where Emil Behring (1854-1917) used Pasteur's methods to develop a vaccine. Impressed by Löffler having achieved immunity in guinea pigs by injecting them repeatedly with small doses of diphtheria bacilli, Behring took a small quantity of serum from one such guinea pig, mixed it with diphtheria toxin and injected the mixture into several animals. To his delight the animals were not harmed. The serum contained a substance that neutralized or destroyed the diphtheria toxin. This was reported in 1890.

About one year later, the first diphtheric child to receive antitoxin was treated in Berlin on Christmas night. It was not until Roux read his classic paper on the subject in 1894, however, that diphtheria anti-toxin began to be used generally. One account of that historic presentation claims:

The staid old scientists, the dignified professors and the sophisticated physicians alike, standing on the seats and throwing their hats in the air, joined in such a noisy and enthusiastic ovation that the safety of the furniture was endangered.

In America William H. Park (1863-1939) was the first outside Europe to develop the diphtheria antitoxin. He did this in 1893. He also definitively established the concept of the carrier of diphtheria. Park and his associate A.L. Beebe concluded, from their study of carriers:

Individuals who have suffered from diphtheria should be kept isolated until cultures prove the bacilli to have disappeared from the throat, for, not only are the bacilli which persist in the throat virulent, but they are not infrequently the cause of diphtheria in others.

Chapin launched a campaign in the 1890s to eliminate diphtheria in Providence, Rhode Island, based on the above results. Bacteriologically tested victims and carriers were isolated. Antitoxin treatment was made compulsory, and a comprehensive program of disinfecting victim's dwellings was carried out. Chapin's aggressive approach to disease prevention soon became the model for public health training and practice in the United States.

Plague Legends

One measure of the speed with which change occurred around that time is seen by the fact that, as late as 1888, J. L. Smith, a clinical professor in New York, still believed that the virus of diphtheria grew in foul, damp places, and that most children developed diphtheria by inhaling infected sewer gas.

Yellow Fever

The 'germ' of yellow fever was not isolated until well into the 20th century. The question of whether to quarantine or not continued to dominate the public health scene throughout the 19th century. Changing ideas concerning how yellow fever spread altered quarantine procedures, as seen from the history of yellow fever in the American south.

Yellow fever never gained ground in Europe, although isolated cases continued to occur following the early epidemics that ravaged Spain and Gibraltar. The northeastern coast of the United States similarly suffered fewer and fewer major outbreaks following those of Philadelphia. In the Southern states of America, however, yellow fever remained the most feared disease throughout the whole of the 19th century. Other diseases caused greater overall mortality but no other disease matched the quickness with which it struck down so many, the horror of the individual deaths that it caused, and the devastating impact it had on commercial life.

Up until around 1840 the belief that yellow fever was a miasmatic and therefore non-contagious disease dominated. This belief more or less paralleled those of the non-contagionists of the European continent, discussed earlier. However, unlike their European counterparts, Southern physicians had the problem of explaining why yellow fever sometimes came and other times did not. Or as one medical editor put it:

> *What a quandary the yellow fever wizards must be in! We have the heat and moisture, dead dogs, cats, chickens, etc., all over the streets, and plenty of hungry doctors; yet Yellow Jack will not come ... How does the present differ from some of the past, in regard to the **peculiar** conditions?*

The idea that yellow fever was carried by individuals and their personal belongings slowly gained ground, receiving strong support by the terrible epidemic of 1853 that started in New Orleans and quickly spread to the cities and towns of Louisiana, Mississippi, and Alabama. While the non-contagionist physicians stood their ground in denying its importation, they no longer disputed *"the fact of transportability as a property belonging to this disease."*

What quarantine measures to adopt depended on the relative importance to be given the sick as carriers of the disease or the physical objects surrounding their movements, i.e. ships, trains, baggage, etc. A vote taken in an 1859 convention chose physical goods over personal contagion by the overwhelming margin of 85 to 6. Rejecting the old system of detention, this convention pushed for the disinfection of ships, baggage, and passengers. Attention turned to which disinfectants were most efficient and effective.

The 1870's saw growing acceptance that yellow fever was caused by a living germ of microscopic size. No longer was yellow fever the product of indigenous filth, heat, moisture or other non-specific factors; it was caused by a transportable poison in the form of a germ. Again the onset of a major epidemic, this time that of 1878, confirmed the new way of understanding the disease. This epidemic was unusual in its ferocity and distribution; it faithfully followed the rail and water lines spreading out of New Orleans, reaching interior towns that had never worried before about yellow fever. Particularly touched were the population that lived closest to railroad stations. Now the vast majority of New Orleans physicians accepted that *"yellow fever is not indigenous there, and that every new epidemic outbreak of it is due to a new importation."*

A microbial basis for yellow fever strengthened the logic of destroying the suspected habitat of the germ. For the towns this meant sanitation, for ships and other means of transport, disinfection. Ship disinfection became so important and so highly organized that some replaced the notion of quarantine with that of 'maritime sanitation'. Incoming vessels were detained for far shorter periods of time; disinfection replaced detention, thereby easing the passage of goods. The apparent success of the new strategy was evident by the fact that New Orleans was free of yellow fever between 1878 and 1897.

The outbreaks that did occur during this period, although small and confined in area, brought to light the persistence of quarantine measures that dated back to the years of the true plague. Armed guards ringed infected towns to prohibit both entrance and exit. Healthy people were locked up in their quarantined houses along with those infected with yellow fever. Certificates of 'good health' were issued to those who remained free of any sign of yellow fever after having spent several days under observation. Trains from infected areas were turned back or prevented from stopping. In some instances, mobs tore up the tracks of the lines particularly incriminated.

Plague Legends

The 1897 epidemic proved to all concerned that the system in place to control the spread of yellow fever simply did not work. Valuable time was lost due to the first hundreds cases having being diagnosed as dengue fever.[73] Quarantine measures were instituted in the coastal vacation town where the first outbreak had occurred, but only after thousands of exposed individuals had left the infected area and returned home. Although mild in comparison to past outbreaks, the panic engendered was in some ways greater than the past due to its greater penetration into the Deep South.

Strictly speaking this account of yellow fever should end here with the close of the 19th century, but the next events followed so closely and they proved immediately crucial for the future of yellow fever control that the reader will forgive me, if I continue just a bit further.

Common knowledge had it that Cuba was the source of most of the incoming cases of yellow fever. When America took control of the island in 1898, following the short-lived war against Spain, William Crawford Gorgas was sent to Havana to clean up that city and rid it of yellow fever. His approach was the classic one of giving it *"a good scouring and a good bath."* On his arrival, yellow fever was at one of its lowest points, so no change could be expected. Instead, what happened was the arrival beginning towards the latter part of 1899 and continuing throughout 1900 of some 25,000 non-immune immigrants from Spain followed by a classic outbreak, one that touched most severely the parts of Havana that had been most cleaned! These were the areas where the new comers sought housing; the older and poorer quarters, occupied by the native population practically all immune, suffered much less.

The idea that yellow fever might be caused by a mosquito had already been vented by the Cuban doctor Carlos J. Finlay in 1881. Unfortunately, Finlay was not able to demonstrate this fact although he tried in hundreds of experiments to transmit yellow fever through the bite of a mosquito. He failed because he was not aware of the fact that infected individuals did not become infective to mosquitoes until a latent period of some ten to fourteen days had passed. Henry R. Carter had discovered this fact in 1898 and it was thus

---

[73] Dengue is a viral disease transmitted by mosquitoes of which *Aedes aegypti* is the most important vector. Epidemic dengue does not seem to have been recognized until 1779.

available to the Special Commission headed by Walter Reed and sent to Havana in June 1900 to investigate the latest outbreak.[74]

Gorgas and Finlay were close friends so Gorgas was fully aware of his mosquito theory. Also, the Commission knew of the most recent demonstration by Ronald Ross that mosquitoes were means whereby malaria was transmitted. As well, they were able to learn first hand from Carter the outcomes of his studies. This helps explain how in but a matter of six months time the Commission was able to confirm the correctness of Finlay's hypothesis, put to rest forever the possibility that yellow fever was a person-to-person contagion, and disprove, as well, the possibility that it could be transported by fomites in the personal belongings of travellers.

There was some hesitancy at first to accept the conclusion of the Commission's report. Long-held beliefs are not easily discarded; Florida, for example, was still clinging around that time to the miasmatic theory of malaria transmission, despite Ross' discovery. Many physicians, while accepting the mosquito as one possible mode of transmitting yellow fever, were not ready to discard their belief that the air or fomites could carry the infection as well.

The first effort to stop an epidemic of yellow fever using anti-mosquito measures, which took place in 1903 in Laredo, Texas, was not successful. It proved difficult to get full cooperation of the public to adopt the necessary measures to rid the area of all breeding sites. The next outbreak occurred in New Orleans in 1905. Local authorities immediately engaged in an all out war against the mosquito and disease transmission. The public was urged to report all suspicious cases so that they could be placed in screened rooms for at least the first three days following the onset of fever; to oil/screen cisterns and other possible breeding areas; and to drain, oil or stock with fish other water receptacles. Violators were jailed. The final tally was 452 deaths resulting from 3,402 cases of the fever. But most revealingly, for the first time in history an epidemic of yellow fever had been stopped **before** the first frost. This would be the last major outbreak of yellow fever in America.

---

[74] By keeping precise records of all visitors of patients sick with yellow fever, Carter was able to conclude that only those visitors who had come later than two weeks after the onset of the disease were stricken with it as well.

Plague Legends

Cholera

The story of cholera in the last decades of the 19th century centers on the pandemic of 1892, the outbreak that had caused more than 8,000 deaths in Hamburg. While England reacted to this pandemic more or less as it had the earlier pandemics of cholera, Hermann M. Biggs, responsible medical officer in the City of New York, took advantage of the situation to introduce new surveillance methods based on Koch's discovery of the cholera vibrio.

Biggs' immediate response was to redouble efforts for cleaning the city and for protecting its food and water supplies. A corps of fifty physicians was retained for special service should the cholera arrive. A circular of instruction on the treatment and prevention of cholera was issued in several languages. Several ships that arrived in New York Harbor having reported cases and deaths were all placed on quarantine. Not a single instance of secondary infection occurred in the City.

Of practical as well as historical importance was Biggs using the cholera threat to convince authorities to establish a Division of Pathology, Bacteriology and Disinfection. It was the laboratory work of this Division that dictated the policies of quarantine and of sanitary measures and was the arbiter on questions of diagnosis. Many years later Chapin described the establishment of this Division as *"perhaps the most important step in modernizing public health practice in the United States."* It was in this laboratory where Park formulated the concept of the diphtheria carrier and developed the first diphtheria antitoxin outside Europe.

As this and the next example illustrate, the germ theory gave public health services a new rationale, one that led in America to the establishment of diagnostic laboratories in every state and in most major cities by the end of the century. Similar developments occurred more slowly in Europe.

Plague

Our last story of change concerns plague, and again is one that extends into the early years of the 20th century. Almost forgotten in Europe, and never seen till then in North America, plague had receded from most of the world until 1896. Then an epidemic at Hong Kong marked the beginning of another great phase of plague activity. Hong Kong quickly became the center of intense study. Almost immediately the organism causing plague was found and cultivated. It was shown that the rat flea from infected rats could transmit the disease. Vaccine of killed organisms were prepared and shown to be effective.

Plague spread quickly to other ports of the Far East, especially Bombay. In the next few years India lost 12 million people. From Bombay and the other ports of India, it fanned out to other parts of the world. It reached San Francisco in early 1900; the federal-run laboratory in that city diagnosed the first case on 6 March in Chinatown. Quickly, the whole of Chinatown was cordoned off, while volunteers sprayed disinfectant, scoured the sewers, and began house-to-house inspection. Almost as quickly, the local press, the Chinese community and California's governor denied the presence of plague in California and control measures were forced to cease.

The campaign led by the press was particularly aggressive. The *Chronicle*, for example, characterized the infected rat-plague link as "*humbug*," claiming that "*this whole germ theory is yet in its infancy.*" Doctors who diagnosed plague were abused; the State Bacteriologist was driven from office. Business interests dominated much of the press as well as the politics both at state and local levels. These interests, particularly those of the all-powerful Southern Pacific Railways, feared restrictive quarantines. To reduce tensions the federal authorities opted for a period of 'secrecy' to give themselves time to confirm more completely the presence of plague and to devise an eradication program that would be acceptable to all parties concerned. The weekly *Public Health Reports* stopped publishing reports from San Francisco in November 1900.

The Quarantine Act of 1893 had placed ultimate authority for quarantine enforcement in America with the Surgeon General. The threat of yellow fever and cholera had played a major role in convincing the United States government that quarantine should be organized along national lines rather than resting only with the states. But, while federal responsibilities had been greatly expanded, federal intervention still rested on cooperation rather than direction. If the City and State Boards of Health did not want to cooperate, federal officials could not intervene. So intertwined were business and political interests that both the California and San Francisco Boards were under continuing pressure to deny the presence of plague and to resist any interventions that could be taken as proof of its presence.

Federal authorities were forced to move slowly, seeking first to build a consensus among public health officials across the country. The question was put before a conference of state boards of health in October 1902; this resulted in the holding of a special plague conference in Washington in January 1903.

Plague Legends

In advance of this conference, the new Governor of California privately conceded the presence of plague to the federal health officials. The conference concluded that the existence of plague in San Francisco had been established beyond doubt, and authorized uniform quarantine restrictions on that city. The whole of California was threatened to quarantine if preventive measures were not quickly put in place. A formal invitation was finally issued on 2 February calling upon the Governor and Mayor to institute a plague-eradication program *"under the supervision of the (federal) Public Health and Marine Hospital Service."* By the end of March, the whole of Chinatown had been inspected, and hundreds of premises sprayed and limed. Old buildings were torn down and unsanitary premises closed down. By June it was possible for federal and California authorities to jointly announce that *"there is no need for quarantine restrictions of travel or traffic to or from that State."*

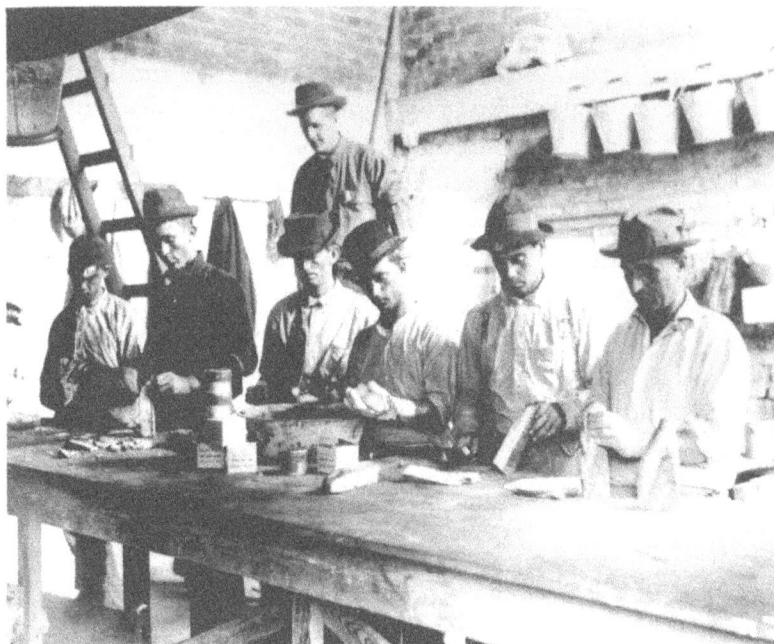

Between 1900 and 1904 some 110 people died of bubonic plague, although authorities believed this was grossly under reported. Almost all victims were Chinese. On 18 April 1906 a massive earthquake struck San Francisco resulting in raging fires that could not be controlled. Chinatown was destroyed and the city's commercial center gutted. Plague reappeared in May 1907, this time spreading throughout the city and into neighboring Oakland. Chinatown had been rebuilt with rat-proof buildings, and as a consequence, very few Chinese died. By the time the epidemic subsided in 1908, there had been 159 cases and 78 deaths reported. Subsequently, plague remained endemic among rats in the bay area, and among squirrels there and in surrounding areas. Plague still exists today among susceptible rodent population in America's sparsely populated west and mid west.

* * * * *

Public health emerged in the 18th and 19th centuries essentially as a humanitarian response to the evidence that poverty and disease went hand-in-hand. The miasmatic theory of disease strongly supported the logic of cleaning up the environment to control epidemic diseases. It was often so loosely constructed as to easily accommodate the reality of a microbe. Only after a more complete picture of the etiology of each individual disease was developed did it become possible to discard once and for all erroneous concepts from the past.

The triumph of the germ theory also led to the discrediting of humoral remedies such as bleeding and purging. It became more and more difficult and finally impossible to argue that one disease could change to another in the course of any given illness, as the specificity of microbial life became well established. The therapeutic goal shifted quickly from one of balancing humors to getting rid of infectious microbes.

Perhaps the most dramatic changes to be made were the establishment of public health laboratories to investigate new outbreaks and the overhauling of the vast institutional structures and administrative arrangements dedicated to quarantine measures, as already hinted at in the examples provided above. However, as seen in these same examples, the new approach to epidemics by and large was not popular. Given a choice, most people preferred not to be inoculated, not to have their homes sprayed or limed, and not to have to undergo periodic physical examinations. The old measures were preferable because they brought about desired changes, even if they were less effective in terms of disease reduction than the new measures. This dilemma still remains present today. In some ways, owing to a more sophisticated public, obtaining their full compliance in the fight against epidemic disease is more difficult to achieve today than ever before, as witness recent efforts to use aerial spraying to control West Nile virus-carrying mosquitoes. But this is a subject for another occasion!

Epilogue

A man may imagine things that are false, but he can only understand things that are true. (Isaac Newton)

So many false things had been imagined in the course of two thousand years of epidemic disease history that the emergence of the truth eventually proved to be a long and drawn out affair. The few truthful insights that did occur before the 18th century were largely ignored, buried and often forgotten. Science, as it is known today, had not yet been borne. Conjectures could come and go with no systematic attempts mounted to prove or disprove them. Those that survived were largely those that ruled by majority vote or by edict, rarely by experimental challenge and verification.

The 18th century faired better in the field of clinical medicine with great advances in anatomy and pathology, but epidemiology still seemed trapped in ancient ideas and beliefs. The domain of study was too great for any real progress to be realized. There were specialists, who appreciated the dilemma they were in, but resources as well as methodological know-how were inadequate for the task, and in many instances required field studies were opposed by medical traditionalists. Only in the 19th century did real progress begin to take place. Once the role of microbes was appreciated, there was no turning back; humoral and miasmatic theories were quietly and relatively quickly buried.

So rapid and dramatic was the progress made, that it was common to believe at the beginning of the 20th century that vaccines would be found for all epidemic diseases and their use would lead to the elimination of most if not all major plagues. As everyone knows today, this did not happen. Only smallpox has been eradicated; all the others are still with us, and in some instances, e.g. plague, malaria and tuberculosis, in more dangerous forms. In fact, the situation for malaria is alarming as it is returning to areas of the world where it had been eliminated earlier in this century. An equally alarming situation is developing for tuberculosis, as it has developed such a high degree of drug resistance as to require the use of multi-drug therapy over a long period of time.

Instead of winning the war against microbes, the human species seem to at best be engaged in a holding action. Not only are some of the oldest disease scourges returning in greater force than ever, many new diseases have emerged as well, for example AIDS, Ebola, hantavirus, and a variant of

Creutzfeldt-Jakob disease (CJD). Intriguingly, these new diseases have generated modern versions of 18th and 19th century controversies, especially concerning the identification of disease-causing agents and the role of environmental change in triggering epidemics.

AIDS, for example, was thought at first by some scientists to be a known disease that was acting with a new factor to create a new disease condition. Syphilis and African swine fever were favored for some time by these specialists even after HIV had been discovered. A more radical position, somewhat paralleling Pettenkofer's belief that Koch's cholera vibrio did not cause cholera, has been that of the virologist Peter Duesberg. He argues that AIDS is not a consequence of infection with HIV but instead of extended exposure to pathogens from illicit drugs or unpurified blood factor VIII. He claims, like Lassis had for yellow fever and plague in the early 1800s, that the disease called AIDS has existed for a long time and only emerged in an epidemic form in the 1980s because of changing life-styles. The scientific community has mocked and vilified Duesberg for his views. There is now overwhelming evidence that HIV infection leads to AIDS. However, it seems that while his views concerning the role of HIV are essentially wrong Duesberg has raised questions concerning the slow progression of the disease and the apparent inactivity of HIV that deserved a better hearing than they received.

A technically more difficult controversy surrounds a group of animal and human diseases now known as spongiform encephalopathies. This group includes scrapie, kuru, Creutzfeldt-Jakob disease (CJD) and its variant, and Bovine Spongiform Encephalopathy (BSE) - Mad cow disease. These diseases involve brain damage and may be inherited, be laterally transmitted through infection, or occur 'spontaneously'. Regions within diseased brains have a characteristic porous and spongy appearance, evidence of extensive nerve cell death; affected individuals exhibit neurological symptoms including impaired muscle control, loss of mental acuity, memory loss and insomnia.

Scrapie, a sheep disease, has been known for over 200 years. It was first seen in England, Scotland and France. The first human spongiform encephalopathy identified is the disease kuru. This disease was found in the late 1950s and occurs among isolated tribal people in the central New Zealand highlands. The origin of the disease is linked to the fact that this tribe mourned their dead by eating some of their brain matter. For a hundred years it had been known that scrapie could be passed on to young sheep by inoculating them with brain tissue from a sheep with scrapie. Now it was found that a disease resembling kuru could be transmitted to different species of primates by inoculating them with human brain biopsy material taken from kuru-suffering patients.

At first it was thought that the disease-causing agent was a slow acting virus, since the incubation period of the disease was long, often many years. The research of Stanley Prusiner, who began his work in 1972 after one of his patients died of CJD, introduced an alternative and totally new agent, one that he named 'prion,' derived from 'proteinaceous infectious particle.' In 1982 he and his colleagues successfully produced a preparation derived from diseased hamster brains that contained a single infectious agent, i.e. prions. The scientific community greeted this discovery with great skepticism; there is still not a consensus whether in fact these particles fully explain this group of new diseases. However, Prusiner continued his research and received the Nobel Prize for medicine/physiology in 1997 for this work.

The issue became more urgent to resolve when new variants of this disease group emerged in cattle in the 1980s and then in humans in 1995. Bovine spongiform encephalopathy (BSE), commonly known as Mad Cow disease, was first identified in southern England in 1985-86. Then in late 1995 two teenagers were diagnosed with CJD, and a further ten cases were announced in April 1996, all unusual in that the age of the patients ranged from nineteen to thirty-nine, well below the normal age associated with CJD. As well, brain pathology revealed excessive amounts of abnormal prion protein lesions. These cases were designated as a new CJD variant. The presence of abnormal prion protein naturally lends support to Prusiner's position, but intensive controversy still rages among scientists engaged in fully explaining these new diseases. Those who believe that a virus or viruses may still be found to play a role are finding it harder to raise the necessary funds to continue their research as available research funds are granted to prion researchers.

Another critical aspect of today's plagues is their intimate link with environmental change. Throughout history this link has been noticed over and over again. In relation to malaria it will be remembered that Lancisi accused Pope Gregory XIII of having made a *"great error"* when he cut down a large wood lying to the south of Rome. Rush expressed concern with how new millponds and the clearing of forestland contributed to bilious and remitting fevers. Also noted, in the history of cholera, is how a volcanic explosion in 1815 triggered off a series of ecological changes that may have led to the emergence of a new and more dangerous form of the cholera vibrio.

Recent research concerning cholera has led to rather dramatic new insights concerning how this disease spreads, ones which may better explain 19th century pandemics than earlier theories. Earlier it had been believed that the cholera vibrio died off quickly in the environment. Now it is realized that cholera can survive in unfavorable environmental conditions in a dormant state and revive when exposed to heat. Cholera bacteria have been found on plankton capable of surviving long voyages in the ocean and reaching areas where the climate is more favorable to its growth. The cholera epidemic that began in Peru in 1990 and spread to 16 other countries in Latin America is thought to have reached the Peruvian coast in a contaminated ship's hull or via contaminated sea plankton.

Among the so-called newly emerging diseases, several examples are worthy of mention to illustrate just how complex is the disease-environment link. An outbreak of Venezuelan hemorrhagic fever in the late 1980s was eventually traced to land-use changes. Chronically infected cotton rats are believed to serve as the source of infection for humans. The clearing of forest improved both the habitats and food sources for rats. The outbreak coincided with a large influx of seasonal agricultural workers needed to work the newly cleared land.

A much earlier outbreak in Argentina of another hemorrhagic fever was linked with the use of herbicides to eliminate weeds among corn crops. While the herbicide eliminated the short weeds, taller grasses were not affected and took over the area where the shorter weed had been previously growing. These grasses provide the food for a rare field mouse whose population at that point exploded. The mouse is a carrier of the Junin virus, the cause of Argentine hemorrhagic fever. The virus is transmitted to humans via the mouse's urine and by dust contaminated with infected rodent excreta.

Many other examples can be added to these. The resulting picture is one of great complexity. The Hippocratic treatise *On Airs, Waters, and Places* would have to be totally overhauled to include the new factors to be taken into account in the study of epidemics. But its underlying message would not need any updating. One might presume that such studies are of central importance in the modern approach to plague prevention and control. Alas, this is not the case. If anything, the divide between field and laboratory research has widened making it more difficult than ever to conduct such studies.

Hippocrates called upon physicians to come to understand the environment to be better prepared to know which diseases were more likely to be present. Today the importance of the environment is found only after outbreaks have occurred. Rarely if ever is such knowledge used to predict and prevent outbreaks, although most reviews of the subject strongly support preventive work. Incentives in the public sector to engage in a better understanding of 'air, water and places' are simply not comparable with the much greater financial rewards to be found in the private sector, where the search concentrates on the development of new disease-preventing vaccines and new disease-treating drugs.

A history of 20th century plague fighting would demonstrate how the epidemic prevention philosophy of the earlier public health movement has lost ground. Perhaps the fact that microbiology and public health in the 19th century grew out of two parallel and largely competing endeavors has proved too great a handicap to overcome. Had the Pasteurian revolution emerged from within existing socially oriented, anti-miasmatic institutions, the history of the 20th century might have been different. But, as we have seen, it did not. Today the split is greater than ever between those who focus only on combating disease-causing agents and those who seek to prevent disease outbreaks by all means available, including social and economic ones. Hopefully, in the 21st century, the human race will develop a public health response to the threat of epidemics that brings together needed field and laboratory disciplines in an effective and efficient manner.

Plague Legends

Acknowledgements

To Susan, my wife, who suggested the title plague legends, and who had to endure far more legends than ended up being included in the final text.

To the late Ken E. Mott who encouraged me to begin this book by lending me books from his personal library.

To J. Barney Frazer, who read and extensively commented on early drafts and my son Steve for his constructive comments and cover design.

To Sandra Hilber Litsios and Vivienne Meyer for their careful proofreading of the final draft.

To Jack Woodall for his suggested corrections and additions to Chapter IV.

To K. Codell Carter for his suggested ammendements to the sections concerning epidemic puerperal fever and Koch's postulates

To the members of the Ficino discussion group, particularly Valery Rees, for advice concerning source references and materials on renaissance and reformation related subjects.

To Paul Russell, who sent me his own handwritten translation of Ficino's plague treatise.

To Edward T. Morman, who brought to my attention the monumental work of August Hirsch.

Remaining faults are those of the author and no one else.

Illustration Credits

Further Reading

Listed below are the books and articles for those wishing to read further on the subject. Those marked with an asterisk (*) proved most useful to me. They were the source of essential ideas, quotes and facts around which this book was created. The references are listed as close to the section where they were used, even when they covered subjects of a much broader nature. Their titles should allow the reader to judge their relevance to other sections of the book as well. Finally, some texts were found on the web; these are noted with an exclamation mark (!). Links to these can be found at the website sciencehumanitiespress.com

General

Ackerknecht, Erwin H *A Short History of Medicine* (Baltimore: Johns Hopkins University Press, 1968)

Baron, AL *Man Against Germs* (London: Robert Hale Limited, 1958)

Cartwright, Frederick F *Disease and History* (New York: Dorset Press, 1991)

Haggard, Howard W *Devils, Drugs and Doctors* (New York and London: Harper & Brothers, 1929)

Hays, JN *The Burdens of Disease: Epidemics and Human Response in Western History* (New Brunswick and London: Rutgers University Press, 1998)

Hirst, L Fabian *The Conquest of Plague* (Oxford: At the Carendon Press, 1953)

Krieg, Joann P *Epidemics in the Modern World* (New York: Twayne Publishers, 1992)

Major, Ralph H *Disease and Destiny* (New York and London: D Appleton-Century Company, 1936)

*Nuland, Sherwin B *Doctors: The Biography of Medicine* (New York and Oxford: Vintage Books, 1988)

Oldstone, Michael BA *Virsuses, Plagues and History* (New York: Oxford Univesity Press, 1998)

Oliver, Wade W *Stalkers of Pestilence: The Story of Man's Ideas of Infection* (College Park, Maryland: McGrath Publishing Company, 1930)

*Porter, Roy *The Greatest Benefit to Mankind: A Medical History of Humanity* (New York and London: WW Norton & Company, 1997)

Riese, Walther *The Conception of Disease: its History, its Versions and its Nature* (New York: Philosophical Library, 1953)

*Riley, James C *The Eighteenth-century campaign to avoid disease* (New York: St Martin's Press, 1987)

Risse, Guenter R Epidemics and Medicine: The Influence of Disease on Medical Thought and Practice *BullHistMed*53:505-519, 1979

Rosen, George *A History of Public Health* (New York: MD Publications, Inc, 1958)

Smith, Geddes *Plague on Us* (New York: The Commonwealth Fund, 1943)

Plague Legends

*Winslow, Charles-Edward A *The Conquest of Epidemic Disease* (Madison, London: The University of Wisconsin Press, 1980)

Wood, George *Wood's Practice of Medicine Vol 1* (Philadelphia: JP Lippincott & Co, 1858)

Chapter I - Ancient Roots of 18th Century Medicine

The Hippocratic Legacy

*!Hippocrates *On Airs, Waters and Places* (translated by Francis Adams and found on the Internet Classics Archives)

*!Hippocrates *Of the Epidemics* (translated by Francis Adams and found on the Internet Classics Archives)

Hippocrates *The Theory and Practice of Medicine* (New York: the Citadel Press, 1964)

The Galenic Legacy

*!Galen *On the Elements According to Hipppocrates* (translated by W J Lewis, with the assistance of J A Beach and S Rubio-Fernaz)

*!Galen *On Hippocrates On the Nature of Man* (translated by WJ Lewis, with the assistance of JA Beach)

*!Galen *On the Natural Facilities* (translated by Arthur John Brock)

Ancient Medicine Shaped by Christianity

!Armstron, A Hilary *St Augustine and Christian Platonism* (The Saint Augutine Lecture 1966)

*French, RK *Robert Whytt, The Soul, and Medicine* (London: The Wellcome Institute of the History of Medicine, 1969)

*Lovejoy, Arthur O *The Great Chain of Being* New York: Harper & Row, Publishers, 1965)

!Plato *Timaeus* (translated by Benjamin Jowett)

Temkin, Oswei *Hippocrates in a World of Pagans and Christians* (Baltimore and London: The John Hopkins University Press, 1991)

Chapter II - Decline of Galenism and the Rise of New Schools of Medicine

Singer, Charles *A Short History of Anatomy & Physiology from the Greeks to Harvey* (New York: Dover, 1957)

Temkin, Owsei *Galenism: Rise and Decline of a Medical Philosophy* (Ithaca, NY: Cornell University Press, 1969)

King, Lester S 'The Transformation of Galenism' in Debus, Allen G (editor) *Medicine in Seventeenth Century England* (Berkeley and Los Angeles: University of California Press, 1974)

The Revolt of Paracelsus

Jacobi, Jolande (editor) *Paracelsus: Selected Writings* (Princeton: Princeton University Press, 1979)

Pachter, Henry M *Magic into Science: The story of Paracelsus* (New York: Henry Schuman, 1951)

Sigerest, Henry E *Paracelsus: Four Treatises* (Baltimore and London: The Johns Hopkins University Press, 1996)

Galen's Anatomy Revisited by Vesalius

Vesalius, Andreas 'Preface to De Fabrica' in *Source Book of Medical History* (New York: Dover Publications Inc, 1960)

Harvey's Explorations of the Heart and Blood

Harvey, William *The Circulation of the Blood and other writings* (London: Everyman's Library, 1990)

Paracelsians and the Iatrochemical School of Medicine

*Debus, Allen G *The English Paracelsians* (New York: Franklin Watts, Inc, 1965)

Rather, LJ 'Pathology at the Mid-Century: A Reassessment of Thomas Willis and Thomas Sydenham' in Debus, Allen G (editor) *Medicine in Seventeenth Century England* (Berkeley and Los Angeles: University of California Press, 1974)

Boyle's Corpuscles and the Iatrophysical School of Medicine

*Boyle, Robert *The Sceptical Chymist* (London & New York: Everyman's Library, 1964)

*Kaplan, Barbara Beigun "*Divulging of Useful Truths in Physick*": The Medical Agenda of Robert Boyle* (Baltimore and London: The Johns Hopkins Press, 1993)

Keele, Kenneth D 'The Sydenham-Boyle Theory of Morbific Particles' *Med Hist* **18**:240-8, 1974

Webster, C 'Water as the Ultimate Principle of Nature: The Background to Boyle's Sceptical Chymist' *Ambix* **XIV**:96-107, 1966

Return to the Hippocratic Bedside

*Dewhurst, Kenneth *Dr. Thomas Sydenham (1624-1689): His Life and Original Writings* (Berkeley and Los Angeles: University of California Press, 1966)

Chapter III - On the Origin of Epidemics

Cipolla, Carlo M *Fighting the Plague in XVIIth century Italy* (Madison: The University of Wisconsin Press, 1981)

*Debus, Allen G *Man and Nature in the Renaissance* (Cambride: Cambridge Univeristy Press, 1978)

Plague Legends

*Jacob, James R *The Scientific Revolution: Apirations and Achievement, 1500-1700* (New Jersey: Humanities Press, 1998)

Mandrou, Robert *From Humanism to Science: 1480-1700* (Middlesex and New York: Penguin Books, 1985)

Siraisi, Nancy G *Medieval & Early Renaissance Medicine: An Introduction to Knowledge and Practice* (Chicago and London: The University of Chicago Press, 1990)

Neo-Platonic, Religious and other 'Occult' Influences

*Craven, JB *Dr Robert Fludd, The English Rosicrucian: Life and Writings* (Montana: Kessinger Publishing Company, 1902)

*Debus, Allen G 'Renaissance Chemistry and the Work of Robert Fludd' *Ambix* **IX**:42-59, 1966

*Ficino, Marsilio *Book of Life* (Woodstock, Connecticut: Spring Publications, 1994)

Ficino, Marsilio *Consiglio contro la pestilentia* (Translated by Paul A Russell

Ficino, Marsilio *Meditations of the Soul: Selected Letters of Marsilio Ficino* (Rochester, Vermont: Inner Traditions International, 1997)

*Hunt, Richard M *The Place of Religion in the Science of Robert Boyle* (Pittsburgh: University of Pittsburgh Press, 1955)

Pagel, Walter 'The Religious and Philosophical Aspects of van Helmont's Science and Medicine' *Bull Hist Med* Suppl No2:44pp, 1944

*Pagel, Walter 'Religious Motives in the Medical Biology of the XVIIth Century' *Bull Hist Med* **3**(2):97-128, 213-31, 265-312, 1935

*Pagel, Walter *Joan Baptista Van Helmont: reformer of science and medicine* (Cambridge: Cambridge University Press, 1982)

Thomas, Keith *Religion and the Decline of Magic* (London, New York and Vienna: Penguin Books, 1971)

Webster, C 'English Medical Reformers of the Puritan Revolution: A Background to the 'Society of Chymical Physitians'' *Ambex* **XIV**:16-41, 1966

*Yates, Frances A *Giordano Bruno and the Hermetic Tradition* (Chicago and London: The University of Chicago Press, 1964)

Germs of Contagion - the Path Least Taken

*Fracastorii, Hieronymi *De Contagione et Contagiosis Morbis et Eorum Curtaione, Libre III* Translation and Notes by Wilmer Cave Wright (New York and London: GP Putnam's Sons, 1930)

*Nutton, Vivian 'The Seeds of Disease: An explanation of contagion and infection from the Greeks to the Renaissance' *Medical History* **26**: 1-34, 1983

Nutton, Vivian 'The Reception of Fracastoro's Theory of Contagion' *OSIRIS*, 2nd series 6:196-234, 1990

On the Epidemic Constitution of the Atmosphere

Goodhall, EW 'A French Epidemiologist of the Sixteenth Century' *Ann Med Hist* 7:409-27, 1935

Chapter IV - Disease Profiles

Burnet, Sir Macfarlane *Natural History of Infectious Diseases* (Cambridge: At the University Press, 1962)

Cox, FEG (editor) *The Wellcome Trust Illustrated History of Tropical Diseases* (London: The Wellcome Trust, 1996)

Desowitz, Robert *Who Gave the Pinta to the Santa Maria?* (New York: WW Norton and Company, 1997)

Fenner, Frank et al *Smallpox and its Eradication* (Geneva: World Health Organization, 1988)

Litsios, Socrates *Influenza and the Work of WHO* (unpublished paper, 1998)

*Major, Ralph H *Classic Descriptions of Disease* (Springfield and Baltimore: Charles C Thomas, 1939)

Zinsser, Hans *Rats, Lice and History: A Study in Biography* (Boston: Little, Brown and Company,1934)

Chapter V - 18th Century - A Kind of Status Quo Reigns

Plague in Marseilles: 1720-22

*Biraben, Jean-Noël Les hommes et la peste en France et dans les pays européens et méditerranéens

England Awaits the Plague

*Baine, Rodney M *Daniel Defoe and the Supernatural* (Athens, Georgia: University of Georgia Press, 1968)

!Browne, Joseph *A Practical Treatise on the Plague* (WHO's on-line historical library)

Burtt, EA *The Metaphysical Foundations of Modern Science* (Garden City, NY: Doubleday & Company, Inc, 1954)

*Defoe, Daniel *A Journal of the Plague Year* (London and Toronto: JM Dent & Sons ltd, 1931)

Nicholoson, Watson *The Historical Sources of Defoe's Journal of the Plague Year* (Port Washington, New York: Kennikat Press, Inc, 1966)

Slack, Paul *The Impact of Plague in Tudor and Stuart England Tuberculosis* (Oxford: Clarendon Press, 1990)

Tuberculosis -The Ignored Ideas of Benjamin Marten

*Dubos, René and Dubos, Jean *The White Plague* (New Brunswick: Rutgers University Press, 1992)

Cotton Mather Battles Smallpox

*Beall, Otho T and Shryock, Richard H *Cotton Mather: First Significant Figure in Americal Medicine* (Baltimore: The Johns Hopkins University Press, 1954)

Cassedy James H *Medicine in America: A Short History* (Baltimore: The Johns Hopkins University Press, 1991)

Plague Legends

Farley, John 'The Spontaneous Generation Controversy (1700-1860): The Origin of Parasitic Worms' J Hist Bio 15(1): 95-125, 1972.

Haggard, Howard W *The Doctor in History* (New Haven and London: Yale University Press, 1934)

Mather, Cotton *On Witchcraft* (New York: Bell Publishing Company)

Shyrock, Richard Harrison *Medicine in America: Historical Essays* (Baltimore: The Johns Hopkins Press, 1966)

*Shyrock, Richard H 'Germ Theories in medicine prior to 1870: further comments on continuity in science' *Clio Medica* 7:81-109, 1972

Diphtheria in the American Colonies: 1736-40

*Caulfield, Ernest 'The Throat Distemper off 1735-1740' *Yale J Bio&Med* 1939

Stannard David E 'Death and the Puritan Child' in *Puritan New England* (New York: St. Martin's Press, 1977)

*Wood W Barry *From Miasmas to Molecules* (New York and London: Columbia University Press, 1961)

Malaria in the Roman Campagna

Bruce-Chwatt LJ and de Zulueta J *The rise and fall of malaria in Europe: A historico-epidemiological study* (Oxford: Oxford University Press, 1980)

*Celli, Angelo *The History of Malaria in the Roman Campagna* (London: John Bale, Sons and Danielson, Ltd, 1933)

Cassedy, James H *Medicine & American Growth: 1800-1860* (Madison: the University of Wisconsin Press, 1986)

*Jarcho, Saul *Quinine's Predecessor: Francesco Torti and the Early History of Cinchona* (Baltimore and London: The Johns Hopkins University Press, 1993)

Typhus in England

Creighton, Charles *A History of Epidemics in Britain* (London: Frank Cass & Co Ltd, 1965)

Influenza - The Views of Arbuthnot and Webster

*Patterson, K David *Pandemic Influenza: 1700-1900* (Totowa, New Jersey: Rowman & Littlefield, 1986)

Yellow Fever in Philadelphia: 1793

Carey, M *Miscellaneous Essays* (New York: Burt Franklin, 1830)

*Powell, John H *Bring Out Your Dead* (Philadelphia: University of Pennsylvania Press, 1993)

Rush's Doctrine of the Unity of Fevers

Bynum WF and Nutton V (eds) *Theories of Fever from Antiquity to the Enlightenment*

*Lawrence, Christopher Cullen, Brown and the Poverty of Essentialism *Med Hist* Suppl No 8, 1-2, 1988

Webster's Views on the Origin of Yellow Fevers

Rosen George 'Noah Webster - Historical Epidemiologist' *J Hist Med* **20**:97-114, 1965
Scott-Warthin Aldred 'Noah Webster as Epidemiologist' *JAMA* **80**: 755-764, 1923
*Webster, Noah *Letters on Yellow Fever Addressed to Dr William Currie* (New York: Arno Press, 1979)

Chapter VI - 19th Century - Recognition of Disease Specificity Opens the Door to Specific Disease Causation

*Ackerknecht Erwin H, 'Anticontagionism Between 1821 and 1867', *Bull, Hist of Med* **22**:562-93, 1948
Hirsch, August *Handbook of Geographical and Historical Pathology* (London: The New Sydenham Society, 1886)
Jones, Martin Owen 'Climate and Disease: The Traveler Describes America *BullHistMed* **41**:254-66, 1967
Wilson, Leonard G Fevers and Science in Early Nineteenth Century Medicine *JHistMed* **33**:386-407, 1978

Broussais Uses Pathological Anatomy to Show All Fevers to Be the Same

*Ackerknacht, Erwin H 'Broussais or a Forgotten Medical Revolution' *Bull Hist Med*, 27:320-43, 1953
Foucault, Michael *The Birth of the Clinic* (New York:Pantheon Books, 1973)
Rolleston, JD 'F.J.V. Broussais (1772-1838): His Life and Doctrines' *ProRoySocMed 32:405-413, 1939*

Distinguishing Typhus from Typhoid Fever

*King, Lester *Transformation in American Medicine: From Benjamin Rush to William Osler* (Baltimore and London: The Johns Hopkins University Press, 1991)
*Gerhard, William W 'On Typhus and Typhoid Fevers' in *Classics in Medical Literature from the University of Pennsylvania* (Philadelphia: Medical Affairs University of Pennsylvania, 1965)

Bretonneau Establishes the Specificity of Diphtheria

*Bretonneau, Pierre *Memoirs on Diphtheria from the writings of Bretonneau, Guersant, Trousseau, Bouchut, Empis and Davot* (London: The New Sydenham Society, 1859)
Rolleston, JD 'Bretonneau: His Life and Work. President's Address' *ProRoySocMed Hist Med,* 1924

Plague Legends

*Trousseau A *Clinique Médicale de L'Hotel-Dieu de Paris* (Paris: J-B Bailliére et Fils, 1865)

Yellow Fever in Europe - To Quarantine or Not?

*Chervin, Nicholas *Examination of the New Opinions of Dr Lassis on Yellow Fever* (Paris, 1829)
*Chervin, Nicholas *Letter to Dr Monfalcon de Lyon on the Yellow Fever that Reigned in Gibraltar in 1828* (Paris, 1830)
Rochoux, Jean-Andre *Dissertation sur Le Typhus Amaril* (Paris: Chez Béchet Jeune, Librairie, 1822)

Cholera Reaches the New World

*Bilson, Geoffrey *A Darkened House: Cholera in Nineteenth Century Canada* (Toronto, Buffalo and London: University of Toronto Prese, 1980)
Le Mée, René Le Choléra et al Question des Logements Insalubres à Paris (1832-1849) *Population,* **1-2**:379-398, 1998
Parkin, John *Disease and Prevention of Disease* (London: John Churchill, 1859)
*Rosenberg, Charles E *The Cholera Years* (Chicago and London: The University of Chicago Press, 1962)

Specific Modes of Transmission for Cholera and Yellow Fever Lost in the 'Sanitary Idea' and Conflicting Causation Theories

Evans, Alfred S Pettenkofer Revisited: The Life and Contributions of Max von Pettenkofer (1818-1901) *Yale J BioMed,* **46**:161-176 (1973)
Himmelfarb, Gertrude *The Idea of Poverty: England in the Early Industrial Age* (London and Boston: Faber and Faber, 1984)
Howard-Jones N Gelsenkirchen Typhoid Epidemic of 1901, Robert Koch, and the Dead Hand of Max von Pettenkofer *BMJ 13 January 1973*
Longmate, Norman *King Cholera: The Biography of a Disease* (London: Hamish Hamilton, 1966)
Pelling, Margaret *Cholera, Fever and English Medicine 1825-1865* (Oxford: Oxford University Press, 1978)
Pickstone, John V 'Death, dirt and fever epidemics: rewriting the history of British 'public health', 1780-1850' in Ranger, T and Slack P (editors) *Epidemics and ideas* (Cambridge: Cambridge University Press, 1992)
Snowden, Frank M *Naples in the Time of Cholera, 1884-1911* (Cambridge: Cambridge University Press, 1995)

Apparent Water, Soil and Air Sources of the Malarial Fever

*Fantini, Bernardino 'Unum facere et alterum non omittere: antimalarial strategies in Italy, 1880-1930' *Parassitologia* **40** (1-2):91-101, 1998.
Flexner, James Thomas *Doctors on Horseback* (New York: Garden City Publishing Co, Inc, 1939)

*Drake, Daniel *Malaria in the Interior Valley of North America* (Urbana, Illinois: University of Illinois Press, 1964)

Duberge, A-P *Le Paludisme* (Paris: Société D'Editions Scientifiques, 1895)

King, Lester S 'The Medical Milieu of Daniel Drake' *JAMA* **254**(15):2126-8, 1985.

Russell, Paul F 'Daniel Drake - Outstanding Pioneer in the Epidemiology of Malaria in America' *Rivista di Parassitologia* **XX**(4):371-8, 1959.

Worboys, Michael 'From miasmas to germs: malaria 1850-1879' Parassitologia **36** (1-2):61-68, 1994.

Epidemic Puerperal Fever - A Hand or Air-Borne Disease?

*Carter, K Codell 'Semmelweis and His Predecessors' *MedHist* **25**:57-72, 1981

*Carter, K Codell 'Ignaz Semmelweis, Carl Mayrhofer, and the Rise of Germ Theory' *MedHist* **29**:33-53, 1985

Lowis, George W 'Epidemiology of Puerperal Fever: The Contributions of Alexander Gordon' *MedHist* **37**:399-410, 1993

Weissmann, Gerald 'Puerperal priority' *The Lancet* **349**:122-25, 1997

Pasteur Takes on Spontaneous Generation

Dubos, René *Louis Pasteur: Free Lance of Science* (New York: Da Capo Press, 1960)

Vallery-Radot, Rene *The Life of Pasteur* (New York: Garden City Publishing Co, Inc)

The Disease Causation Postulates of Koch

*Carter, K Codell 'Koch's Postulates in Relation to the Work of Jacob Henle and Edwin Klebs' *MedHist* **29**:353-74, 1985

Microbial Approach to Public Health

Chambers, JS *The Conquest of Cholera: America's Greatest Scourge* (New York: The Macmillan Company, 1938)

*Humphreys, Margaret *Yellow Fever and the South* (New Brunswick: Rutgers University Press, 1992)

Litsios, Socrates William Crawford Gorgas (1854-1920), *Perspectives in Biology and Medicine* (with the editor)

*Mayne, Alan *The Imagined Slum: Newspaper Representation in Three Cities 1870-1914* (Leicester, London and New York: Leicester University Press, 1993)

*Mullen, Fitzhugh *Plagues and Politics:TheStory of the United States Public Health Service* (New York: Basic Books, Inc, Publishers, 1989)

Epilogue

Garett, Laurie *The Coming Plague* (New York and London: Penguin Books, 1994)

Plague Legends

*Oldstone, Michael BA *Viruses, Plagues & History* (New York and Oxford: Oxford University Press, 1998)

WHO *Health and Environment in Sustainable Development: five years after Rio* (Geneva: World Health Organization, 1997)

Index

Addison, Joseph, 115, 116

Aetius, 84

AIDS, 229, 230

Alchemy, 27, 75

Amulets, 54, 62, 63

Anatomy, anato-pathology, 29, 154, 155, 238, 239, 243

Animalculae, 114, 116

Arbuthnot, John, 110, 113, 114, 132, 133, 134, 242

Aretaeus, 84, 86

Aristotle, 9, 12, 16, 17, 18, 25, 31, 35, 36, 37, 42, 61, 68, 205

Asclepiades, 12, 13, 15, 16, 48

Astrology, 19, 51

Athens, Great Plague of, 11, 80

Atmosphere, 3, 7, 8, 9, 13, 15, 16, 26, 36, 38, 47, 52, 53, 56, 57, 58, 59, 64, 65, 67, 68, 70, 71, 72, 73, 74, 75, 79, 83, 90, 95, 101, 107, 108, 109, 110, 111, 112, 113, 125, 126, 129, 130, 131, 133, 134, 135, 136, 137, 138, 141, 143, 145, 150, 151, 153, 164, 169, 173, 174, 175, 179, 181, 182, 183, 186, 187, 188, 191, 193, 194, 195, 197, 198, 199, 202, 203, 205, 207, 209, 210, 214, 217, 219, 223, 233, 240

Atomic or corpuscular theory of disease, 12, 13, 43, 48, 63, 71, 109, 112

Avicenna, 25

Baglivi, Giorgio, 46

Baillou, Guillaume de, 71, 72

Bard, Samuel, 85

Bassi, Agostino, 202

Behring, Emil, 219

Bentham, Jeremy, 185

Bichat, Xavier, 154, 155, 156, 157, 207

Biggs, Hermann M, 224

Bile, bilious, yellow and black, 9, 79, 84, 111, 127, 128, 137, 140, 146, 193, 231

Black Assizes, 130

Blood, 13, 32, 33, 91, 119, 203, 239

Boerhaave, Hermann, 141, 142, 143, 144

Boissier de Sauvages, François, 78, 93

Bologna, University of, 53

Bonetus, Theophilus, 154

Borelli, Gian Alphonso, 46, 48

Boyle, Robert, 43, 44, 45, 48, 62, 64, 71, 72, 73, 75, 106, 118, 134, 151, 205, 206, 239, 240

Boylston, Zabdiel, 120

Braun, Carl, 201, 202, 203

Bretonneau, Pierre-Fidèle, 84, 85, 86, 161, 165, 166, 167, 169, 170, 176, 210, 243

Broussais, François, 153, 154, 156, 157, 158, 159, 160, 161, 166, 170, 243

Brown, John, 141, 142, 143, 144, 156, 157, 158, 159, 170, 192, 241, 243

Browne, Joseph, 111, 112, 113, 115, 241

Budd, William, 163, 164, 165, 183, 185, 188

Buffon, Comte de, 145

Carter, Henry R, 222, 223, 245

Casaubon, Meric, 57

Celsus, Cornelius, 89

Chadwick, Edwin, 182, 185, 186

Chapin, Charles V, 217, 219, 224

Charles II, 22

Charles V, 32, 217

Chemistry, 23, 27, 37, 43, 44, 101, 142, 143, 240

Chervin, Nicolas, 172, 173, 174, 176, 244

China, 80, 127, 133, 151

Cholera, 95, 97, 175, 176, 182, 185, 186, 187, 224, 232, 244, 245

Cole, William, 46

Comets, 106

Contagion, contagious, 4, 10, 16, 66, 67, 68, 69, 70, 71, 85, 92, 104, 107, 109, 110, 112, 113, 114, 117, 123, 129, 135, 138,

139, 143, 144, 147, 149, 150, 163, 164, 165, 167, 168, 169, 172, 173, 174, 176, 178, 179, 182, 187, 188, 189, 198, 199, 201, 202, 211, 217, 221, 223, 240
Copernicus, Nicolas, 18, 43
Cordon Sanitaire, 102, 103, 110, 175
Creutzfeldt-Jakob disease (CJD), 230
Cullen, William, 93, 141, 142, 143, 144, 163, 243
Currie, William, 148, 149, 150, 151, 243
Dante, 24
de Vinci, Leonardo, 31
Defoe, Daniel, 105, 108, 113, 114, 139, 241
Democritus, 48, 71
Demon, demonic, 21, 29, 30, 54, 58, 116, 142
Dengue, 222
Descartes, René, 35, 36, 43, 61, 78, 205
Devèze, Jean, 171
Diet, 8, 27, 65, 111, 114, 135, 141, 143, 145, 155, 158, 199
Diphtheria, 10, 71, 84, 85, 101, 113, 119, 122, 123, 124, 125, 146, 147, 160, 166, 167, 169, 182, 216, 218, 219, 224
Dissection, 14, 29, 30, 31, 35, 154, 155
Divine wrath and punishment, 3, 120
Drake, Daniel, 94, 178, 191, 192, 193, 194, 195, 196, 198, 245
Drug(s), 14, 21, 144, 229
Duchesne, Joseph, 42, 61
Duesberg, Peter, 230
Edinburgh, as center of medical education, 22, 85, 93, 142, 143, 144, 161, 163, 198
Elliot, George, 160
Emmerich, Rudolph, 189, 190
Encyclopedia Brittanica, 128
England, 22, 33, 43, 44, 60, 61, 77, 78, 80, 82, 85, 87, 93, 95, 105, 110, 112, 118, 123, 128, 130, 142, 146, 147, 149, 158, 162, 175, 176, 183, 186, 217, 224, 230, 231, 238, 239, 241, 242, 244
Enlightenment, 101
Environment, 24, 43, 101, 145, 150, 214, 217, 227, 232, 233

Epidemic constitution, 4, 10, 16, 36, 42, 47, 58, 60, 71, 72, 73, 74, 75, 126, 129, 133, 135, 176, 182, 183, 187, 188, 190, 191, 193, 194, 195, 196, 197
Fabrizio, Giralomo, 33, 34
Farr, William, 186, 187, 188
Ferments, fermentation, 39, 63, 107, 112, 114, 116, 197, 206
Fever(s), 10, 40, 41, 46, 48, 52, 69, 71, 73, 75, 77, 80, 81, 82, 87, 88, 89, 90, 92, 93, 94, 95, 98, 99, 100, 103, 104, 123, 125, 126, 128, 129, 130, 131, 137, 138, 139, 140, 141, 143, 145, 146, 148, 149, 150, 151, 156, 157, 160, 161, 162, 163, 164, 165, 170, 171, 173, 174, 182, 185, 187, 188, 190, 191, 193, 194, 195, 196, 198, 199, 200, 202, 203, 218, 220, 221, 222, 223, 230, 232, 244
Ficino, Marsilio, 2, 17, 20, 24, 52, 53, 54, 55, 56, 57, 74, 240
Fludd, Robert, 4, 23, 57, 58, 59, 60, 61, 62, 63, 75, 101, 116, 240
Fomites, 67, 68, 70, 87, 109, 129, 223
Fothergill, John, 85
Fracastoro, Girolamo, 4, 32, 65, 66, 68, 69, 70, 94, 101, 117, 240
France, 3, 29, 37, 57, 71, 82, 85, 96, 101, 103, 105, 110, 126, 137, 151, 152, 155, 158, 162, 170, 173, 175, 176, 197, 205, 215, 217, 230, 241, 242
Galen, 7, 11, 12, 13, 14, 15, 16, 17, 18, 20, 21, 24, 25, 29, 30, 31, 32, 33, 34, 35, 41, 43, 47, 51, 56, 61, 65, 69, 88, 154, 155, 238, 239
Gassendi, Pierre, 43, 60, 61
Gerhard, William Wood, 160, 161, 162, 163, 243
Germs, 4, 65, 66, 67, 68, 69, 70, 72, 76, 116, 120, 181, 188, 191, 197, 202, 206, 207, 208, 209, 211, 245
Gilbert, William, 62, 63
Gordon, Alexander, 198, 203, 245
Gorgas, William, 222, 223
Guaiac, 26, 56, 127
Hales, Stephen, 131

Harvey, William, 22, 23, 32, 33, 34, 35, 36, 41, 46, 58, 60, 142, 154, 205, 238, 239

Heart, 32, 33, 239

Henle, Jacob, 201, 202, 211, 212, 245

Hermes Trismegistus, Hermetic, 2, 53, 54, 57, 58, 59, 60, 61, 63, 64, 75, 93, 183, 240

Hippocrates, 1, 3, 4, 7, 8, 9, 10, 11, 12, 14, 15, 16, 17, 19, 21, 24, 29, 31, 46, 47, 51, 53, 54, 65, 66, 68, 71, 72, 74, 81, 82, 84, 88, 99, 101, 109, 118, 127, 128, 142, 145, 150, 155, 191, 233, 238

Hirsch, August, 153, 187, 196, 197, 243

Hobbes, Thomas, 3

Holmes, Oliver Wendell, 119, 147, 158, 159, 198, 199, 203

Howard, John, 130, 131, 217, 237, 242

Humor(s), humour(s), 115

Humor(s), humour(s),, 8, 9

immunity, 91, 170, 222

Immunity, 87, 91, 169, 170, 189, 216, 219

Infection, infectious, 64, 66, 67, 99, 101, 109, 113, 135, 143, 150, 151, 160, 161, 164, 202, 227, 231, 237

Influenza, 90, 132, 135, 153, 169, 241, 242

Insects, as carriers of disease, 93, 94, 95, 115, 119, 126, 151, 196

Italy, 21, 24, 29, 53, 85, 96, 102, 116, 127, 155, 167, 189, 196, 239, 244

Jenner, Edward, 121, 216

Jenner, William, 162

Keats, John, 84

Kepler, Johannes, 60, 62

Kircher, Athanasius, 64, 111, 118

Klebs, Edwin, 197, 211, 214, 218, 245

Koch, Robert, 117, 160, 188, 189, 190, 211, 212, 214, 215, 216, 217, 218, 219, 224, 230, 244, 245

La Mettrie, 155

Laënnec, René, 158

Lancisi, Giovanni Maria, 125, 126, 231

Lassis, S, 172, 230, 244

Laveran, Alphonse, 196, 197

Leeuwenhoek, Antony van, 114, 116, 119, 205, 206

Lesions, 86, 98, 157, 161, 162, 215, 216, 218, 231

Liebig, Justus von, 187, 201, 206, 207

Lind, James, 129, 130, 131, 198, 217

Lister, Joseph, 210

Liver, 8, 18, 30, 31, 32, 89, 94, 139, 207

Locke, John, 47, 116, 154

Löffler, Friedrich, 218, 219

London, plague in, 113

London, Royal Society of, 114, 118, 205

Louis, Pierre, 158, 160, 161, 163, 173, 174, 186

Louvain, University of, 29

Lucca, anti-tuberculosis legislation, 117

Lungs, 22, 25, 32, 33, 79, 90, 92, 114, 115, 119, 134, 183, 197, 215

Macrocosm/microcosm, 55, 57, 58, 61, 116, 238

Magnetism, 60, 62

Malaria, 10, 77, 88, 89, 125, 126, 128, 145, 151, 152, 157, 162, 191, 193, 194, 195, 196, 197, 202, 211, 214, 218, 223, 229, 231, 242, 245

Marryat, Frederick, 145

Marten, Benjamin, 114, 115, 116, 119, 241

Mather, Cotton, 115, 118, 120, 123, 241

Mather, Increase, 118

Mayrhofer, Carl, 202, 203, 211, 245

Mead, Richard, 108, 109, 110, 111, 112, 113, 118, 135, 217

Measles, 10, 48, 59, 74, 77, 87, 91, 123, 148, 150

Mercury, 25, 26, 27, 47, 56, 72, 208

Mersenne, Marin, 60, 61, 62

Metchnikoff, Elie, 189

Methodist school of medicine, 48

Methodist School of Medicine, 12

Miasma(s), 3, 144, 153, 175, 186, 187, 190, 191, 199, 202

Microscope, 34, 64, 93, 107, 111, 116, 195, 207

Milne, AA, 148
Montaigne, 80
Moon, 18, 51, 108
Morbid, morbific matter, 3, 7, 8, 40, 73, 136, 146, 151, 156, 162, 165, 166, 181, 182, 191, 197, 203, 211
Morgagni, Giovanni Battista, 154, 155
Mosquitoes, 89, 94, 95, 126, 170, 197, 198, 222, 223, 227
Needham, John T, 205
Newton, Isaac, 75, 106, 108, 142, 144, 205, 229
Occult, 4, 20, 23, 36, 42, 54, 58, 60, 61, 68, 71, 73
Odor(s), 63, 64, 68, 85, 95, 107, 126, 137, 169, 182, 201, 207
Oertel, MJ, 218
Osler, Sir William, 42, 134, 162, 243
Oxford, University of, 44, 237, 241, 242, 244, 246
Padua, as center of medical education, 29, 30, 32, 33
Pandemic(s), 90, 91, 92, 95, 96, 97, 133, 135, 151, 160, 169, 175, 190, 215, 224
Paracelsus, 4, 22, 23, 24, 25, 26, 27, 29, 36, 37, 38, 39, 40, 42, 44, 45, 47, 51, 56, 57, 60, 77, 118, 144, 176, 238, 239
Pariset, Etienne, 172
Park, William H, 219, 224, 237
Parkin, John, 182, 244
Pasteur, Louis, 3, 4, 158, 160, 198, 201, 202, 203, 204, 205, 206, 207, 208, 209, 210, 211, 214, 215, 216, 217, 219, 245
Pathology, 40, 46, 155, 156, 157, 160, 208, 229, 231
Patin, Guy, 35
Pestilence, 16, 20, 80, 113, 135, 138, 140, 149, 181, 182
Petit, Marc-Antoine, 161
Pettenkofer, Max von, 1, 183, 187, 188, 189, 190, 191, 197, 208, 215, 230, 244
Pfeiffer, Richard, 215, 216
Phlegm, 8, 9, 14, 42
Pitcairn, Archibald, 46

Plague, 2, 3, 4, 5, 10, 16, 19, 51, 52, 54, 59, 63, 64, 66, 70, 71, 74, 78, 79, 80, 82, 92, 101, 102, 103, 104, 105, 106, 107, 108, 109, 110, 111, 112, 113, 115, 116, 119, 125, 133, 143, 147, 150, 151, 164, 172, 178, 189, 191, 199, 202, 217, 218, 221, 224, 225, 226, 229, 230, 232, 233
Planets (Jupiter, Venus et al), 18, 51, 52, 54, 57, 58, 69, 70, 106
Plants, 53, 56, 58, 64, 195, 196, 211
Plato, 2, 17, 18, 21, 51, 53, 55, 238
Plotinus, 18
Pneuma, 15, 32, 33, 35
Pope Gregory XIII, 126, 231
Pope Innocent XI, 125
Pope Pius VI, 128
Pores (body), 12, 33, 34, 35, 45, 46, 65, 67, 107, 124
Pouchet, Félix Archimède, 208, 209
Pringle, Sir John, 131
Prusiner, Stanley, 231
Public health, 5, 186, 189, 190, 208, 217, 218, 219, 220, 224, 225, 227, 233, 244
Puerperal fever, 48, 198, 199, 200, 201, 202, 203, 207, 211
Putrefaction, 67, 68, 69, 70, 71, 111, 137, 165, 183, 195, 200, 206, 207, 208, 209, 210
Pye, George, 110, 113
Quarantine(s), 76, 80, 102, 110, 135, 150, 172, 175, 176, 177, 178, 179, 188, 189, 220, 221, 224, 225, 226, 227
Quinine, 47, 48, 88, 144, 192
Redi, Francesco, 205
Reed, Walter, 223
Rhazes, 52, 81
Rosicrucians, 61, 75
Ross, Ronald, 197, 223
Roux, Emile, 219
Royal Society, 42, 114, 118, 205
Rush, Benjamin, 1, 95, 114, 134, 137, 138, 139, 140, 141, 142, 143, 144, 145, 146, 147, 148, 150, 151, 152, 153, 158, 170, 192, 231, 242, 243
Russell, Paul F, 10

Salt, 25, 26, 38, 41, 42, 109, 114, 179
Salve, 62, 63
Sanarelli, Giuseppi, 216
Scarlet fever, 48, 87, 101, 123, 125
Scrapie, 230
Scrofula, 63, 82
Semmelweis, Ignaz, 245
Serres, Etienne-Renaud-Augustin, 161
Servetus, Michael, 22
Shakespeare, William, 82, 90
Smallpox, 10, 74, 77, 80, 81, 98, 101, 118,
    119, 120, 123, 124, 153, 164, 165, 168,
    169, 202, 216, 229
Smith, Nathan, 163, 164
Snow, John, 182, 183, 184, 185, 187, 189
Soil, 176, 183, 187, 188, 190, 191, 193, 194,
    195, 196, 197
Soul, 17, 18, 24, 25, 29, 32, 35, 36, 55, 78
Spain, 84, 85, 90, 96, 116, 117, 170, 172,
    220, 222
Spallanzani, Lazzaro, 205
Spleen, 8, 10
Spontaneous generation, 63, 64, 69, 121,
    205, 206, 207, 208, 209, 210
Sulfur, 25, 26, 27, 41, 42, 47, 125
Sun, 18, 51, 57, 58, 70, 108, 116, 126, 135,
    138, 175, 195
Swift, Jonathan, 110, 134
Sydenham, Thomas, 4, 44, 47, 48, 72, 73,
    74, 77, 87, 92, 116, 118, 129, 134, 142,
    143, 145, 149, 151, 154, 239, 243
Sylvius, Franciscus, 40
Sylvius, Jacobus, 31, 40, 41, 47, 48
Syphilis, 26, 37, 56, 65, 80, 101, 127, 156,
    202
Therapeutics, treatment, 7, 8, 11, 12, 19,
    22, 25, 26, 37, 39, 40, 47, 61, 63, 72, 124,
    126, 139, 140, 141, 143, 144, 156, 157,
    160, 166, 167, 178, 191, 219, 224
Thucydides, 11, 88, 147
Tommasi-Crudeli, Corrado, 197, 214
Torti, Francesco, 126, 242

Trousseau, Armand, 157, 159, 166, 170,
    173, 174, 243, 244
Tuberculosis, 10, 16, 48, 59, 66, 67, 68, 77,
    82, 83, 84, 85, 114, 115, 116, 117, 145,
    212, 214, 216, 218, 229
Typhoid, 10, 48, 77, 85, 98, 153, 157, 160,
    161, 162, 163, 164, 165, 166, 183, 185,
    187, 188, 189, 190, 193, 217, 218
Typhomalaria, 162
Typhus, 66, 77, 92, 93, 94, 98, 128, 129, 130,
    138, 143, 145, 146, 161, 162, 163, 165,
    170, 173, 202, 217, 218
Universal Soul, 18
Vallisnieri, Antonio, 121
van Helmont, Jean Baptiste, 4, 23, 37, 38,
    39, 40, 44, 45, 48, 57, 60, 62, 63, 64, 101,
    118, 240
Velpeau, Alfred, 166, 167, 176
Vesalius, Andreas, 22, 29, 30, 31, 32, 33,
    155, 239
Villermé, Louis René, 174
Virchow, Rudolf, 207, 208, 217
Walpole, Horace, 125
Water, 8, 9, 10, 13, 26, 36, 37, 38, 41, 44, 52,
    57, 59, 63, 70, 97, 98, 113, 125, 133, 135,
    136, 140, 141, 143, 146, 170, 183, 184,
    185, 186, 187, 189, 190, 191, 194, 196,
    197, 205, 208, 221, 223, 224, 233
Webster, Noah, 112, 113, 114, 132, 133,
    134, 135, 147, 148, 149, 150, 151, 152,
    161, 163, 164, 172, 182, 193, 239, 240,
    242, 243
Whooping cough, 71, 72, 123
Whytt, Robert, 78, 238
Willis, Thomas, 36, 41, 42, 46, 47, 48, 92,
    98, 118, 161, 239
Winds, 9, 58, 60, 70, 109, 126, 133, 136, 147,
    174, 182, 187, 191
Winslow, Charles Edward A., 1, 2, 4, 238
Wood, George, 85, 146, 158, 161, 181, 182,
    238
Wren, Christopher, 98

Yellow fever, 1, 4, 76, 94, 95, 101, 134, 137, 138, 140, 145, 146, 147, 148, 150, 151, 164, 170, 171, 172, 173, 174, 176, 177, 178, 179, 189, 191, 216, 217, 218, 220, 221, 222, 223, 225, 230

Yersin, Alexandre, 219
Zinsser, Hans, 160, 241
Zymotic theory of disease, 207

Also by Socrates Litsios

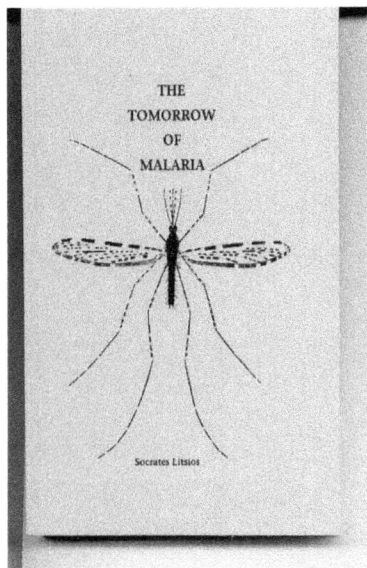

Previous publications include the prize winning book *The Tomorrow of Malaria* published in 1996 and numerous historical articles published in professional journals, including Perspectives in Biology and Medicine, Medical Anthropology, and Parassitologia.

What reviewers had to say about Litsios' The Tomorrow of Malaria

Winner of 1996 Pacific Prize awarded by Pacific Press.

"Thought provoking and an excellent review."
(Abram S. Benenson in Journal of Public Health Policy)

"A fine powerful little book."
(Robert S. Desowitz in Nature)

"Required reading for all who would understand the history of malaria during the past century and for those who plan the malaria campaigns during the next."
(Margaret Humphreys in Journal of the History of Medicine)

"Immensely readable."
(Mary J. Dobson in Medical History)

"Potent and captivating."
(Mary R. Galinski in Parasitology Today)

"Rare artistry as well as scholarship."
(Chev Kidson in Southeast Asian Journal of Tropical Medicine and Public Health)

"A little gem of a pocket book."
(M.W. Service in Annals of Tropical Medicine and Parasitology)

The Tomorrow of Malaria can be purchased at the NHBS web site, www.nhbs.com

Plague Legends

Books from Science & Humanities Press

HOW TO TRAVEL — A Guidebook for Persons with a Disability — Fred Rosen (1997) ISBN 1-888725-05-2, 5½ X 8¼, 120 pp, $14.95

HOW TO TRAVEL in Canada — A Guidebook for A Visitor with a Disability — Fred Rosen (2000) ISBN 1-888725-26-5, 5½X8¼, 180 pp, $14.95

AVOIDING Attendants from HELL: A Practical Guide to Finding, Hiring & Keeping Personal Care Attendants 2nd Edn — June Price, (2001), paperback edition (2001) ISBN 1-888725-60-5, 8¼X6½, 200 pp, $18.95

The Bridge Never Crossed — A Survivor's Search for Meaning. Captain George A. Burk (1999) The inspiring story of George Burk, lone survivor of a military plane crash, who overcame extensive burn injuries to earn a presidential award and become a highly successful motivational speaker.   ISBN 1-888725-16-8, 5½X8¼, 170 pp, illustrated. $16.95

24-point Gospel — The Big News for Today – The Gospel according to Matthew, Mark, Luke & John (KJV) in 24-point typeType is about 1/3 inch high. Now, people with visual disabilities like macular degeneration can still use this important reference. "Giant print" books are usually 18 pt. or less ISBN 1-888725-11-7, 8¼X10½, 512 pp, $29.95

Me and My Shadows — Shadow Puppet Fun for Kids of All Ages - Elizabeth Adams, Revised Edition by Dr. Bud Banis (2000) A thoroughly illustrated guide to the art of shadow puppet entertainment using tools that are always at hand wherever you go. A perfect gift for children and adults. ISBN 1-888725-44-3, 7X8¼, 67 pp, 12.95

Growing Up on Route 66 — Michael Lund (2000) ISBN 1-888725-31-1 Novel evoking fond memories of what it was like to grow up alongside "America's Highway" in 20th Century Missouri. (Trade paperback) 5½ X8¼, 260 pp, $14.95

Route 66 Kids — Michael Lund (2002) ISBN 1-888725-70-2 Sequel to *Growing Up on Route 66*, continuing memories of what it was like to grow up alongside "America's Highway" in 20th Century Missouri. (Trade paperback) 5½ X8¼, 270 pp, $14.95

MamaSquad! (2001) Hilarious novel by Clarence Wall about what happens when a group of women from a retirement home get tangled up in Army Special Forces. ISBN 1-888725-13-3 5½ X8¼, 200 pp, $14.95

Virginia Mayo — The Best Years of My Life (2002) Autobiography of film star Virginia Mayo as told to LC Van Savage. From her early days in Vaudeville and the Muny in St Louis to the dozens of hit motion pictures, with dozens of photographs. ISBN 1-888725-53-2, 7x10 200 pp, $18.95

Sexually Transmitted Diseases — Symptoms, Diagnosis, Treatment, Prevention-2nd Edition – NIAID Staff, Assembled and Edited by R.J.Banis, PhD, (2006) . Illustrated with more than 70 diagrams and photographs of lesions, ISBN 1-888725-58-3, 8¼X6½, 298 pp, $18.95

The Stress Myth -Serge Doublet, PhD (2000) A thorough examination of the concept that 'stress' is the source of unexplained afflictions. Debunking mysticism, psychologist Serge Doublet reviews the history of other concepts such as 'demons', 'humors', 'hysteria' and 'neurasthenia' that had been placed in this role in the past, and provides an alternative approach for more success in coping with life's challenges. ISBN 1-888725-36-2, 5½X8¼, 280 pp, $24.95

To Norma Jeane With Love, Jimmie -Jim Dougherty as told to LC Van Savage (2001) ISBN 1-888725-51-6 The sensitive and touching story of Jim Dougherty's teenage bride who later became Marilyn Monroe. Dozens of photographs. "The Marilyn Monroe book of the year!" As seen on TV. 5½X8¼, 200 pp, $16.95

Plague Legends: from the Miasmas of Hippocrates to the Microbes of Pasteur-Socrates Litsios D.Sc. (2001) Medical progress from early history through the 19th Century in understanding origins and spread of contagious disease. A thorough but readable and enlightening history of medicine. Illustrated, Bibliography, Index ISBN 1-888725-33-8, 6¼X8¼, 250pp, $24.95

The Job — Eric Whitfield (2001) A story of self-discovery in the context of the death of a grandfather.. A book to read and share in times of change and Grieving. ISBN 1-888725-68-0, 5½ X 8¼, 100 pp, $14.95

Science & Humanities Press

Publishes fine books under the imprints:

- Science & Humanities Press
- BeachHouse Books
- MacroPrint Books
- Heuristic Books

Science & Humanities Press
PO Box 7151
Chesterfield MO 63006-7151
sciencehumanitiespress.com
phone 636-394-4950
Fax 636-394-1381

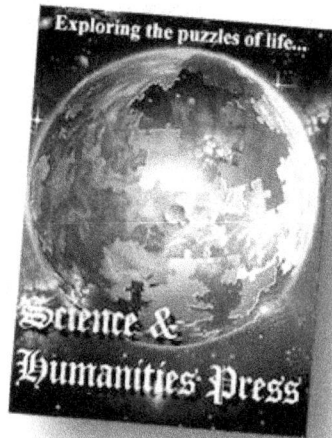

Plague Legends: from the Miasmas of Hippocrates to the Microbes of Pasteur- Socrates Litsios D.Sc. (2001) ISBN 1-888725-33-8 Medical progress from early history through the 19th Century in understanding origins and spread of contagious disease. A thorough but readable and enlightening history of medicine. Illustrated, Bibliography, Index 7.44X9.69, 270pp. $24.95

Watch for new books from Science & Humanities Press at

www.sciencehumanitiespress.com

Order form		Each	Quantity	Amount
Item		Each	Quantity	Amount
Missouri (only) sales tax 6.925%				
Postage & Handling				$5.00
		Total		
Ship to Name:				
Address:				
City State Zip: